A Cure 4 Dieting

Your Body Changes...
So Should How You Lose Weight

DR. RICHARD (RICK) HENNINGSEN

Just Because
Something Is Done,
Doesn't Mean It's
What Should Be Done!

Library of Congress: CN-1-7183577704

Cover Design: Jessica James – Pro_designx

Copy Editor: Carole Berglie

Publisher: Hasmark

ISBN 13: 978-1-989161-50-0
ISBN 10: 1989161502

Hasmark PUBLISHING

"So many people I know and love spend years on the "Yo-Yo" diet. Their weight is constantly up and down. Well now, Dr. Rick Henningsen's, **A Cure 4 Dieting** provides the keys to owning your results – not just renting them. I can't wait to share this wisdom with everyone I love."

– Lennox Cornwall, author *Embracing Failure: Your Key to Success."*

"*Most people are approaching weight loss in an ineffective way; causing them to yo-yo on their weight, or worse, gaining more weight than before they started their so-called diet. My recommendation is to dive into this book and you will discover the true cure for long-term and desirable results. The secret to permanent weight loss is finally revealed in this extraordinary piece of work. Follow every word and you will be thrilled that you did.*"

– Peggy McColl, *New York Times* Best Selling Author

"*Lose weight and restore health to every cell of your body while gaining something far more important: Freedom. Be prepared to enjoy a spectacular new zest for life and healthy body-mind-spirit that is now free from the shackles that society and biology has held you in for far too long.*"

– Trace Haskins, CEO, The Awesomeness Company

"*Dr. Rick has provided an exciting new approach to ending the weight loss struggles of millions. He has combined science based advice with inspiration and practical ideas to lead you on your own journey for sustained weight loss.*"

– David Riklan, Founder-SelfGrowth.com

"*Whatever you need to know about obesity and metabolic disease is in **A Cure 4 Dieting**. It is easy to read and if you have a history of struggling with weight you will be clinging onto every word because it tackles the complexities of weight gain to optimize your results. **A Cure 4 Dieting** provided me with more knowledge and tools to continue helping my patients with weight-related challenges. It is the missing piece of the weight loss puzzle. If you, or someone you care about, suffers from seemingly hope-less obesity and metabolic disease, you must read this book! It will change your life too.*"

– Dr. Jussi Eerikäinen, Cardiologist, Mathematician and Neuroplasticity Researcher.

To all those who possess inside themselves the desire,
and the drive, to live an active, healthy lifestyle
free from the restrictions of overweight and obesity.
For dieters everywhere, I offer this information to
help speed you on your way, in your pursuit of...

The Perfect You

Contents

Acknowledgments

I am a firm believer that there is always room for improvement, a smarter way for each of us to achieve the results we desire in life through the understanding and application of knowledge.

I've been fortunate in my life to have attracted a group of incredibly talented mentors. Business men, women, entrepreneurs, and industry leaders. Self-made individuals who themselves learned that in order to succeed, one must not only learn but also apply that which they've learned correctly – and purposefully.

They are the Bob Proctors, Arthur Agatstons, Peggy McColls, Ed and Caroline Cederquists, Mike Dillards, Harold Katz's, Anik Singals, Natalie Ledwells, Jean Evelyn Nidetchs, Loren Cordains, and Fred Lams of the world. The names may or may not be familiar to all, but each possesses the power to transform lives.

They are remarkable leaders and lifelong students, committed to learning, understanding, and applying that which improves the results we achieve in all aspects of life. And each, in his or her respective field, has touched the lives of millions. A special thanks to you – my mentors.

To the team behind *A Cure 4 Dieting*, the publishers, editors, graphic designers, and web developers. This journey would not be possible without your tremendous efforts and support.

To the trial recipients, from the United States, Canada, and Europe, who through application of the contents contained within have achieved extraordinary results, I wish to offer my most sincere gratitude and appreciation for urging me to share this information with the world. I am, as always, honored to be of service to you.

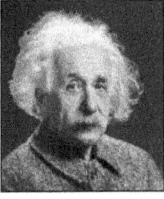

To the memory of Albert Einstein, and all those who through the pursuit of knowledge have empowered the world, and motivated me to discover a better way through the observation, study and research of that which goes unaddressed by traditional weight loss, and dieting strategies. It is true...

"We cannot solve our problems with the same thinking we used when we created them."

And to those of you who through the wise application of the information contained between the covers of this book will embrace the active, healthy lifestyle you desire and deserve.

Preface

Absorb, and purposefully apply, the information contained within the pages to follow. Do so, and you will be amazed at what you can accomplish in as little as a few short days, and weeks. The information on these pages is that powerful.

The Body Changes and So, Too, Must How You Lose Weight

What if one day you were to wake up and learn that all your weight-loss efforts were in vain, that any success you achieved was now destined to reverse itself unless you continued on that course of restricted caloric intake, and eliminating the foods you used to enjoy before your diet?

What if you learned that your short-lived success, as well as your weight-loss failures were not because of an inability to commit to a particular diet or program, but were in fact due to protective mechanisms that are triggered as soon as your body starts to release fat? And what would you do if you learned that the weight-loss strategies or diet plans you were employing were actually responsible for triggering a physiological response in your body to store fat, rather than release it?

Would you continue to use those strategies? Of course not! Now, what if I were to tell you that, if you continue to read on, today would be the day when all that changes? When you would discover the means to ending your weight loss struggles, and make dieting, a thing of the past.

Your inner monologue might kick in and say, "That's impossible. If that were true, I'd would know about it." On the other hand, this suggestion might spark your natural curiosity to investigate something that goes against all you've come to know about weight loss and dieting.

As I sat down to write this book, it dawned on me what I needed to do to help you. I'm going to share with you information that will challenge many of the things you believe about dieting – information that, when applied purposefully, can transform your waistline, and your life, as quickly as it has mine. It is that missing piece of the weight-loss puzzle, a means to an end of lengthy, restrictive weight-loss and dieting strategies – and the key to freeing yourself from a lifetime of fruitless struggles.

As I started to write, another thought came to mind. It was something my mentors have taught me. "We attract into our lives those things which we are ready for." This means, right now, you are supposed to have this information in front of you because you attracted it. You're ready to receive it. Not the author, nor the book; it's the information contained in the pages to follow.

I urge you: *do not* flip through the pages quickly, searching for bits and pieces of information to improve your existing weight-loss efforts. And then close the pages, figuring you "got it." To do so will help improve your results, but it will do little in the way of aiding you to maintain the *results* of your weight-loss efforts. Instead, make a commitment to yourself to absorb, understand, and apply the content within, in its entirety. This information has the power to transform not only your waistline but also every other aspect of your life; and it will change the way you look at weight loss and weight stabilization forever.

Once you fully understand, and wisely apply, the content of this book to your own circumstances, you will discover a new sense of your own self, a confidence that comes with achievement, and a freedom to enjoy all you desire, without the restrictions of overweight and obesity.

You will have a deeper understanding of the mechanisms by which we gain weight. You will learn how to address the changes, blocks, and barriers that interfere with your ability to quickly release unwanted pounds and inches. And you will learn what has eluded dieters for the better part of a century: *how to maintain a healthier weight and waistline indefinitely.*

Your belief system will change as you come to understand how the body and mind respond to weight loss and dieting, and you will understand how to optimize your body's natural ability to process and assimilate the foods you consume, turning them into fat-burning energy to achieve your own extraordinary results.

Now, before I introduce you to the information contained in the pages to follow, allow me to go back and tell you where this information comes from. Just over twenty years ago, my life took a dramatic turn. A career-ending injury, and subsequent surgery, left me sedentary and gaining weight. And like most people gaining weight, I sought out the latest and greatest weight-loss strategies available. I followed the diets. I employed them to the letter. And as advertised, I lost some weight – but then something unexpected happened. I gained all the weight back, and more!

This process repeated itself over the course of five long years. It didn't matter how healthy I thought I was eating, or how much I restricted my dietary intake. Once my diet of the moment came to an end, the weight came back with a vengeance. I was beside myself with frustration. I was under the impression that diets were supposed to help people lose weight, and get a bit healthier. Was I mistaken? Or did I just buy into the hype? Never having been a subscriber to the "*that's the way it is*" mindset, I wanted to know Why? Was is me? How and why did this happen? And more importantly, How Can I Fix It?

These questions set me on a fifteen-year journey of researching some of the most commonly used weight-loss and dieting strategies so I could discover what works, what doesn't, and why. It's a journey that continues to this day. In short, the information that follows will take you far beyond the myopic strategies of reducing your caloric intake below that of your energy expenditure.

This touches upon the physical, psychological, genetic, and environmental factors affecting your weight circumstance, with the goal of increasing your understanding of how the body responds to weight loss and dieting, and of providing you with a means to accelerate, and improve the results of your efforts, and bring an end your weight-loss struggles.

What was once curiosity has become a lifetime quest to improve the results and longevity of the results achieved through our weight loss efforts, but that is not nearly as important as it is for you to understand this information, and apply it correctly to your particular circumstance.

Live well, live long, and enjoy all that life has to offer!

Introduction: Freedom

When I first started to organize the information shared in **A Cure 4 Dieting**, I looked inside myself for the word I felt would best describe the content to follow – a word that would offer readers the power to change their lives. And the word that repeatedly came to mind was: *Freedom*.

Freedom is a powerful thing. It is a state of existence that may be applied to many aspects of life. It is the ability to act, think, or speak without influence, whether that influence be internal or external. It is the ability to experience life without the encumbrance of circumstance that would hold you back – or otherwise keep you where you are.

The freedom I speak of has eluded dieters for the better part of a century. Few dieters will ever experience the freedom of being able to enjoy all foods sensibly, without having to worry about their waistlines or having to diet permanently. It's not because of a dieter's inability to follow through with the weight-loss and dieting strategies but, rather, because the way we are shown to lose weight only affords us the ability to inefficiently manage our weight, and waistlines – and Not to Control It!

I have made it my mission to provide you with exactly that: a means of *controlling* your weight circumstance, so you too can experience this freedom for yourself.

Discover the Freedom

Overweight and obesity are Silent Thieves, stealing those things in life that are most precious to us – time, memories, health, joy, happiness, and the freedom to experience all that life has to offer.

I've been fortunate to have lived on both sides of the fence, going from fit and healthy, to morbidly obese in a few short years. You might ask why I thought this was fortunate, and the answer would be: I was fortunate because, having lived with being overweight and obese, I can see the issues dieters face; I have the eyes of someone who has lived the experience first-hand – something that many weight-loss, diet, and fitness gurus preaching radical lifestyle changes have not and will never experience or understand.

I was fortunate because the particular circumstance of my struggle with obesity afforded me the opportunity to discover the crucial short-comings of weight-loss, and dieting strategies – strategies employed by dieters the world over. And I was fortunate because, without having had this experience, I would never have discovered how to easily address these shortcomings – and achieve the extraordinary results I did in half the time.

The circumstance of my weight issues may differ from yours, but the end result, and the effects of being overweight or obese, are the same for us all. The larger we become, the more we withdraw from experiencing what life has to offer. And the less and less we are able to enjoy the fun, food, and activities that are such a part of this journey we call life.

We enter a realm that is alien to those who have never lived with being overweight or obese. It's a world where health, energy, and the passion for life plummets. Where agility becomes awkwardness, and fear of embarrass-ment stifles the desire to participate in those activities we once so enjoyed, let alone experience new ones. It's a place where even the simplest things can become a struggle.

There is a quote that best described how I felt while I was struggling with obesity. It was used by actor Tim Robbins in his portrayal of banker Andy Dufresne, in speaking to "Red," played by Morgan Freeman in the 1994 movie *The Shawshank Redemption*:

"Get busy living, or get busy dying."

These words resonated with me, mostly I think because I was dying inside. Every time I said no to an invite to participate in something I knew I would have enjoyed, declining because my weight circumstance was holding me back, another little piece of me died inside.

We Are Meant to Thrive in Life, Not Simply Exist

To live to our fullest potential, and enjoy all the human experience can provide, it is up to us to decide how we face life and those challenges that come our way. We can either act to create the changes we desire in life, or through inaction, live with the oppression that overweight, and obesity brings to life.

I sided with Mr. Dufresne, deciding to "get busy living," and to do whatever was necessary to take control of my body, and once again enjoy an active, healthy lifestyle. It was to regain my passion for life, and live life on my own terms free from the restrictions of overweight and obesity.

The task I committed to was an arduous one, and I cannot say with certainty that I would have made that commitment at the time had I known its course would span better than twenty years. It would have been far easier to follow the herd, and spend the rest of my life jumping from one weight-loss strategy to another, hoping this time it would last. But I can say now, without a shadow of a doubt, that I would do it again in a heartbeat, because…

What I found at the end of the journey was far more than a healthier weight and a trimmer waistline. Instead, it was being able again, more than once, having the choice to say "Yes" (or "No") to fun activities and new experiences based solely upon my level of interest – not because my weight circumstance dictated what I could and could not do. That discovery was even better than knowing I'd never have to worry about my waistline – or permanent weight gain, ever again.

It was a renewed sense of self, a confidence that comes from being – and feeling – the best you. It's waking up with energy, ready to take on the day. And it's that feeling you get when you look in the mirror, and smile at what you see.

The goal was not to find a secret pill, a miracle potion, or the next weight-loss plan. It was to learn those things that would improve upon and extend the results achieved with an existing weight-loss strategy, without having to starve in order to do so.

It was about understanding the mechanisms of weight gain – those things that contribute to dietary lifestyle choices. And it was about under-standing why the results achieved through most weight-loss and dieting efforts are short-lived, why we begin to gain weight as soon as we transition from a 'diet' back to a normal routine. And that's regardless of how conscious we are being as to the quantity and nutritional value of the foods we're consuming. Above all, it was about learning how to address those factors that interfere with lasting weight-loss success. I never would have imagined, during the course of my research, that I would stumble upon the missing piece of the weight-loss puzzle. Even now, it is the one thing that remains unaddressed by an entire weight-loss industry.

There are products, plans, and programs that, through the employment of their particular weight-loss strategies, touch upon one, possibly two aspects of the bigger picture. And there are others outside of weight loss and dieting that address other aspects of it. But as a whole, these singularly focused approaches fall short of providing the lasting results that dieters desire, and deserve.

A Cure 4 Dieting provides all who struggle with weight issues a greater understanding of the mechanics of weight gain, its causative agents, and the factors that interfere with the body's ability to lose weight or to maintain a healthy weight and waistline. It provides a means of addressing those factors which interfere with our ability to effectively, and efficiently, manage our weight.

Here is a look at weight loss, and weight stabilization, from a different perspective – an alternative to the singularly focused strategies of "eat less, and exercise more," as well as all those "eliminate this food, and/or eat only that food" – standard strategies that dominate the marketplace.

The content herein will inform, educate, and challenge what you have come to believe about weight loss and dieting, and will introduce you to the benefits of "Optimization" as opposed to "Restrictive" weight-loss and dieting strategies alone. You will discover the pitfalls inherent to dieting, and why dieting is responsible for promoting post-diet weight gain, as well as cyclical dieting.

We cannot solve our problems with the same thinking we used when we created them!

– Albert Einstein

The quote commonly attributed to the great mind of Albert Einstein is a reminder for us to take a step back, to move away from the dieting mentality that has dominated the weight-loss market for the past hundred years. You need to think outside of the box, examining your weight circumstance and taking an accounting of your successes, your failures, and all you've endured to shed those unwanted pounds and inches. You need to correct that which has left you wanting.

There is a tremendous difference between that which provides temporary relief of a particular circumstance, symptom, or condition – in this case your waistline – and that which works toward correcting the issues responsible for causing that circumstance, symptom, or condition. The latter provides an enduring solution, a means to cure or otherwise correct or improve the root cause of a circumstance, symptom, or condition. The former addresses only the circumstance, symptom, or condition, without consideration of the underlying cause.

My wish for you, as you read and absorb the information contained in this book, is that you step back and away from what you have been led to believe about weight loss and dieting, so that you discover that which interferes with your ability to lose weight and maintain a healthy waistline, and you can act purposefully with focus to improve, correct, solve, or otherwise cure the underlying cause of your weight circumstance.

It is only by understanding, and properly applying this information that we may all empower ourselves to escape the self-perpetuating cycle of weight gain and dieting, and we can begin to enjoy life with purpose, on our own terms…

Knowledge is Freedom!

Author's Note

The principles and information in this book will benefit all that apply it to their life's circumstance. It is not just a means to improve upon your ability to lose and maintain a healthier weight and waistline. It is also the means to improve the efficiency by which your body can process and assimilate the foods you consume.

From conception to death, the body is in a constant state of change, and it requires essential nutrients to develop, grow, and repair damaged tissue, replace cells, and maintain normal bodily functions, including providing the energy we need to be active.

The body is incredibly efficient in turning those raw materials, or the foods we ingest, into everything we need to function. However, *times change, food sources change, and so do our bodies*. In order to maintain a healthy weight, normal energy levels, and optimal functionality, we need to address these changes.

Those struggling with weight issues can accelerate, and improve, the results of their weight-loss efforts, as well as learn how to easily maintain a healthy weight and waistline while enjoying all foods sensibly. Others will derive maximum benefit from the foods they consume by optimizing their body's ability to process and assimilate those foods into the essential nutrients to provide the energy the body requires to function at peak levels. And parents will discover a way to instill healthy new eating behaviors in their children.

The past century has witnessed dramatic changes in the foods we produce, grow, and raise. We consume genetically modified food products and processed foods that by law need contain only a small percentage of the whole foods for which they are named. The fruits and vegetables we buy have been sprayed or otherwise exposed to chemicals, pesticides, fertilizers, and environmental pollutants, as well as often irradiated to kill harmful bacteria and parasites.

The animal products we consume come from animals that are fed or injected with hormones and antibiotics. Environmental pollutants and toxins in the air we breathe, the water we drink, and the food we ingest can affect our bodies on a cellular level, and negatively impact the natural balance of our gut biome and digestion. All these things and more contribute to degrading the body's ability to process and assimilate the foods we consume.

Despite their negative effects that the use of these chemicals and antibiotics may have on us, they are a necessary measure to protect us and our food sources from harmful bacteria, pathogens, and parasites. The use of hormones in our foods is an entirely different story.

As times continue to change, our bodies and the foods we eat will continue to be affected by environmental factors, so we too must change and adapt our dietary lifestyle to derive maximum benefit from those foods we do consume, and to minimize the effects of daily exposure to the increasing number of environmental factors that can affect our bodies.

Absorb, understand, and apply this information to your life's circumstance, and you will discover the freedom to live the active, healthy lifestyle you desire, and deserve.

A Cure 4 Dieting

Part I

1

The Truth Is...

We cannot solve a problem with the same thinking that
created the problem to begin with.

– Albert Einstein

There is a freedom that comes from knowing you never have to worry about your waistline – or permanent weight gain ever again, for that matter. There's a confidence and a renewed sense of self in knowing you have conquered your weight issues, and have put an end to your weight-loss struggles, all on your own terms. There is the freedom of knowing you can enjoy all the fun, foods, and activities life has to offer, because you want to and not because your diet or weight circumstance dictates what you can and cannot do.

This freedom comes with the peace of mind of knowing you will never again have to pay for the privilege of subjecting yourself to weeks, or months, of restricted caloric intake and avoidance of foods that make your life more enjoyable.

It is a freedom all dieters seek, but few will ever find. The freedom to enjoy life without compromise. To live without the limitations associated with being overweight or obese, and without the restrictions or radical lifestyle changes imposed by weight loss or dieting strategies employed in a vain attempt to achieve such freedom.

I discovered this freedom not through dieting but despite dieting. The truth is that few people struggling with weight issues will ever find the freedom I'm speaking of if they use dieting alone. That's not because of one's inability to commit to a particular weight-loss strategy, but because the weight loss and the dieting strategies employed by dieters contribute to the very problem they profess to help dieters overcome – weight gain.[1]

The freedom I'm speaking of is available to all seek it, and to achieve it takes no more effort than understanding how to address those things that interfere with your ability to lose and maintain a healthier weight and waistline.

Knowing is ... the new body, face, and mind of weight loss

You're Not in Control

When I first discovered the truth about weight loss and dieting, it challenged everything I believed to be true about how we were taught to lose unwanted pounds and inches, and maintain a healthier weight. I had just spent five years cycling through diet after diet, trying to lose the ten pounds I gained following a career-ending injury and subsequent surgery, and now, five years later, the ten pounds I originally set out to lose were well over forty pounds.

I had spent thousands of dollars on diet foods, products, and supplements following some of the latest and greatest weight-loss and dieting strategies, which I thought were supposed to help me lose weight and keep it off. But all I had to show for my efforts were the years of constant hunger and the constant cravings from restricting caloric intake, avoiding the foods I enjoyed most, not to mention an empty wallet and growing frustration and contempt for my circumstance.

Along with my growing frustration came questions – lots of them. What was I doing wrong? Was it me? Was I just buying into the dieting hype, or was I genetically predisposed to being overweight? Why did I gain all the weight back, and why did I gain even more weight every time I lost weight – even when I was counting calories and watching everything I was consuming? Why didn't my results last? And how come it was getting harder to lose weight every time I began another round of dieting? Was I eating too much? Too little? Was I eating the wrong foods? What was it? *Why was this happening?*

The one thing I was certain of at the time was, I had little to no control over what was happening with my weight. As soon as my diet came to an end, and I transitioned back to a "normal" lifestyle, the results I worked so hard to achieve reversed and the weight piled back on. It didn't matter that I was watching everything I was eating, or that I was eating only twice, sometimes once per day. The weight I lost found me again, and it brought friends.

My existence during those five years reminded me of the movie *Groundhog Day*, with Bill Murray, except I was living the dieting version. No matter what I did in the days or weeks prior, I always ended up right back where I started – a little heavier, a little more confused, and even more frustrated, trying to bring the madness to an end.

Adding insult to injury, I started the dieter's blame game. I began to blame myself for failing to achieve the long-term results I was working so hard to attain. "If I'm watching what I eat, counting calories, and avoiding the foods everyone knows makes us fat, then it must be me!" Diets help people lose weight, so it must be something I'm doing wrong. I began to question everything I was eating – maybe I shouldn't have eaten this or that, as if one moment of indulgence was responsible for reversing weeks or months of hard-earned results.

Then the excuses came. "I must have a slow metabolism." "It's my age, people gain weight as they get older." "It's genetics." I thought, *I don't have the ability to exercise. It's just the way I'm supposed to be. I have my* (insert family member's name here) *body*. But I realized these were nothing more than lies I was telling myself, rationalizations to explain a situation I was unhappy about, I didn't understand, and I had no control over. Or so I thought.

Never being a "That's just the way it is" type of person, I set out to find the answers to my questions and take control of my weight circumstance. And it wasn't long before I found what I was looking for.

There were dozens of articles on the pros and cons of dieting, and why diets don't work, some from a physical perspective, others from an emotional or psychological perspective, but they didn't answer all of my questions. So, I dug deeper, and I found more answers. And the more answers I found, the more questions I had. The rabbit hole went deeper and deeper, and thus began a fifteen-year journey away from dieting and into research, and testing some of the most common types of weight-loss and dieting strategies to find out what really works, what doesn't, and why.

What I discovered is here. This book was written to empower you with the knowledge, tools, and skills to help you optimize the results of your weight loss and stabilization efforts, and to discover the freedom I speak of. It approaches weight loss and dieting from a different perspective.

As you read, you will discover the pitfalls inherent in traditional weight-loss and dieting strategies. You will learn of the barriers that block your ability lose and maintain a healthy weight. And you'll find out how to knock those barriers out of your way, to optimize your body's utilization of its required nutrients.

This is a learning process designed to accelerate the results achieved through your weight-loss efforts, without the need for diet foods, products, caffeinated supplements, dangerous medications, or appetite suppressants. Most important, it shows you how to easily maintain your hard-earned results. And it can be done with no more effort than what you do to lose weight now, with one big exception.

Once you absorb, understand, and apply this information to your life's circumstance, you will never have to worry about your waistline, or permanent weight gain ever again, or the need to spend weeks, or months dieting for results that have proven themselves to be temporary at best.

You will understand how your body responds to weight loss and dieting, and how to manage your waistline with an accuracy you've never known before. You will have the information and tools you need to help you live the active, healthy lifestyle you desire, and deserve, and you will under-stand why – Knowing is the New Body, Face, and Mind of Weight Loss.

Important Things to Know

Earlier I mentioned that the paradigms and beliefs you have regarding weight loss and dieting will be challenged. The beliefs we have, and the practices we employ to lose weight are things we have been taught over time, and they are responsible for the preconceived notions we have about weight loss and dieting. Understanding what they are, and how they influence your weight loss, as well as your stabilization efforts, will help to improve your results.

Beliefs are the trust, faith, and confidence you have in something you believe to be true. It is your acceptance of something as fact, with or without evidence to support those beliefs. Your beliefs, regardless of whether they are founded in facts, will influence your actions and decisions equally.

Our beliefs become the voice of reason guiding our thoughts and actions. They're that little voice inside your head telling you something is either right or wrong, good or bad, safe or dangerous, possible or not possible, and that voice is based upon your life's experience and observations.

Dieting is a perfect example of a firmly embedded belief shared by people the world over. We all know and believe that dieting is what we do when we have to lose weight. You know this to be true without the need for evidence to support this belief, because it is something you've been taught your entire life through friends, family members, at school, by doctors, and from the endless stream of advertisements telling you that what you need to do is diet if you want to lose weight. But just because something is done, doesn't mean it's what *should* be done.

Yes, dieting will help you lose weight, but what most people don't know is that dieting is responsible for triggering protective mechanisms in the body that cause us to gain weight. It is self-perpetuating. It promotes post-diet weight gain and cyclical dieting,[2] which is one reason why the typical dieter finds the need to attempt to lose weight as many as four, or five times every year.[3]

So, where do our beliefs come from? They are the culmination of everything we experience, observe, and learn from the moment we're born. They are those things taught to us by our mothers, fathers, teachers, and preachers that we accept as truth because we learned them from trusted sources and recognized authority figures.

We do not question the validity of the lessons, nor whether the information is correct, fact-based, or even applicable to today's lifestyle. We simply accept them as truth. But the lessons taught to us by our recognized authority figures are not the only way we develop the beliefs we carry in life. They also develop as a result of personal experience, and those things we observe in our environment whether we are consciously aware of them, or not.

It may be difficult for some to grasp, but our beliefs are not always our own, nor are they always true or in our best interests. Earlier, I mentioned that our beliefs also come from the observation of those things we see and hear in our environment, and this is true even if we are not consciously aware of what we are observing.

Our brains process upward of four hundred billion bits of information each second, but we are only capable of being consciously aware of two thousand bits of information per second.[4] This means that billions of bits of information are being processed and stored by our minds without our even knowing it. This leaves plenty of room for us to develop familiarity and acceptance of information we are unconsciously exposed to on a repetitive basis. It's called conditioning.

You've heard of subliminal messaging. Subliminal messages come to us below the level of conscious awareness, and according to vocabulary.com,[5] you shouldn't worry about it, because you will never consciously know you are being conditioned, programmed, manipulated, or controlled unless someone tells you. Consider yourself told.

Subliminal messages are visual and auditory cues often used in advertising to unconsciously heighten the persuasiveness of the advertisement. It can be used with equal effectiveness in conveying a completely different message than what you believe you are seeing or hearing.[6]

You may have experienced an unconscious belief at one time or another when something comes up with which you have had no prior experience, but you nevertheless have an opinion on how that something should be handled. For example, there is never a shortage of those who have never had a weight issue or have never been on a diet in their lives telling us the best way to lose weight.

The key to ensuring that your beliefs are healthy and current is to question them as they arise. If you believe something should or shouldn't be done, ask yourself *why* you believe this, and then listen to the answers. In doing so, you will discover if your belief in something is factual, correct, and true, or if it is false or based on some antiquated notion passed along to you that has no place in or application to today's day and age.

A *paradigm* is a typical set of standards by which you do something. These are learned behaviors often passed down from generation to generation through ritual, tradition, and routine. An example of a paradigm would be eating three square meals per day. This is done in many countries around the world, despite decades-old evidence suggesting that eating three square meals per day is not the most efficient way for people to get the steady supply of nutrients and energy their bodies require throughout the day.

Today, eating three times per day is simply a social convention we've adopted that interestingly enough appears to have been born out of greed and envy, and not because of the body's dietary needs.

Another paradigm practiced by dieters the world over is that of restricting caloric intake, or counting calories, when they want to lose a few pounds and inches. It is the standard on which an entire industry has been built, and it remains a cornerstone of modern-day weight-loss and dieting strategies, despite research suggesting that dieting on its own promotes post-diet weight gain and cyclical dieting.

Paradigms are those things we do without question or thought, *but just because something is done, doesn't mean it's what should be done.*

A good example of how paradigms can be passed from generation to generation comes from the "Holiday Ham Story." Little Jessie was helping mom prepare the holiday ham for dinner. Eager to learn everything there was to know about this holiday favorite, Jessie asked, "Mom, why do you cut the end of the ham off before putting in the pan?"

Jessie's mom thought for a moment, and replied. "I don't know, honey, it's just the way I learned to do it. Why don't you ask grandmother,"

Jessie ran into the next room, and asked, "Grandma, why do we cut the end of the ham off before we put it in the pan?" Grandma thought for a moment, and said, "I have no idea. Let's ask Nana."

The curious trio made their way over to Nana, and asked, "Why do we cut the end of the ham off before we put it in the pot?" Nana thought for a moment, and started to chuckle. "You're still doing that? My mother did that because we couldn't afford a pan big enough to fit the whole ham in, and I did it because using that pan reminded me of her during the holidays."

As simple as this story may seem, the takeaway is this: we develop beliefs and paradigms both consciously and unconsciously, whether or not they are true, necessary, or applicable to present day life. In the case of the holiday ham, the inability to purchase a larger roasting pan was responsible for establishing the paradigm, unquestioned until a curious fifth-generation child noticed it.

Another takeaway from this story is that it is good to question your actions and beliefs as they arise. Why am I doing this? Is there a better way? It's a good way to clean out the misinformation and antiquated beliefs that may be influencing your actions, and causing you to make decisions despite their no longer having value, benefit, or application. Had little Jessie not questioned the reason why her mother cut the end of the ham off while Nana was still around to solve the mystery, the holiday ham paradigm born of necessity five generations earlier would continue to be the practice passed along to future generations, believing that this is just how it's done.

Preconceived notions are the opinions formed beforehand that are based on your beliefs. An example of a preconceived notion would be the first thought that comes to mind after reading the following statement:

You can lose weight faster by eating more, and exercising less.

In this example, it wouldn't be hard to guess that your preconceived notion was, "That's not possible.'" Or it might be something along the lines of, "Wishful thinking!'" That's because this statement challenges what you've been taught to believe your entire life. And this is where the danger lies.

If your preconceived notion was, "It's not possible," you run the risk of dismissing the statement as untrue or having no merit, without questioning or investigating the veracity of the statement. In this case, that would have cost you the opportunity to save time, money, and effort, because the statement is, in fact, 100% true.

It is not only possible to lose weight faster by eating more often than prescribed by the most commonly used weight loss and dieting strategies, but extraordinary results can be achieved with, or without exercise – as you will discover in the pages to follow.

A Hard Pill to Swallow

On occasion, the time comes when we discover something we trusted, accepted, or believed to be true is in fact not what we believed it to be. And learning the truth behind that which we have come to trust and believe in can be a hard pill to swallow. Such was the case for me with dieting.

One of the most disturbing pieces of information I came across in my research was, without a doubt, the hardest pill to swallow: *Dieting is directly responsible for triggering post-diet weight gain, and supports cyclical dieting and the continued need to diet.*[7] I found it strange that this information has existed for years, yet few if any dieters are aware of it, and no one I am aware of in the weight-loss field has ever attempted to find out how to address what is, without doubt, the biggest problem in weight loss and dieting.

As disturbing as this news was to hear for the first time, it makes all the sense in the world. It in part explains the dismal results offered by the most commonly used weight-loss and dieting strategies. It also explains why the average dieter will make multiple attempts to lose weight every year.[8] But it raises more questions than it answers.

Anyone can lose weight even employing the simplest of strategies. People do it all the time. But why can't they keep it off? Depending on which source you cite, only 1 to 5% of dieters will ever succeed at losing and maintaining a healthy weight and waistline, which means *upwards of 99% of dieters will fail* at achieving lasting results.

This may seem like bad news, and if you are among the 1 to 5% of those who have achieved long-term success through dieting, it likely is bad news, because achieving long-term success with traditional weight-loss and dieting strategies alone requires the willpower to live with the restrictions and compromises associated with them.

I can't imagine anyone wanting to live the remainder of his or her life in a state of constant hunger, restricting caloric intake, watching every morsel of food put into the mouth, counting calories, and avoiding the foods enjoyed most – just to maintain a smaller waistline – that's unless your livelihood depends on it. Fortunately, there's no need to. Even those of you willing to live a life of compromise to maintain your weight and waistline will discover – there is a better way.

The truth is, dieting to lose weight is much like taking your car to the carwash for a tune-up. It'll look good for a while, but it does nothing to improve what's going on under the hood, which is exactly where dieters need to focus if they wish to lose weight and maintain a healthier weight and waistline without the restrictions and compromises.

Now, if you are one of the 99% of dieters struggling with weight issues, and you are reading this, this is fantastic news. You are about to discover the reasons behind your weight loss and stabilization struggles, and learn how to address them without the need for diet foods and all those other products designed to artificially boost your metabolism or suppress the appetite.

In the past, you may have held the misconception that you were in control of your weight circumstance because of your ability to go on a diet when you want to lose a few pounds and inches, but the truth is that you can't control what you don't know about, nor can you control what you don't understand.

Dieting, by the very nature of what it is and how it is done, can only offer temporary results to those who use dieting alone as a means to lose weight. Restricting your caloric intake, as is done with dieting, causes physiological changes in the body that are responsible for reversing the results achieved from your weight-loss efforts once your diet comes to an end. This makes dieting nothing more than an inefficient way to manage your weight and waistline. It is something that comes with a cost far beyond the money you spend on diet foods, products, and supplements.

There Is a Better Way

In order to improve the efficiency and effectiveness of your weight loss efforts, you must understand the mechanisms behind weight gain and how dieting and weight loss affect the body. It is only by knowing this that you can take control of your weight and address those things that interfere with your ability to lose weight, as well as maintain a healthier weight and waistline. *Knowing* is the first step to achieving the lasting results you desire, and deserve.

Chapter Summary

- Just because something is done, that doesn't mean it's what should be done!

- Knowing is the New Body, Face, and Mind of Weight Loss.

- You cannot efficiently manage your weight through dieting alone.

- Paradigms are the standards by which something is done.

- Preconceived notions are opinions based upon our beliefs.

- Your beliefs, right or wrong, influence your actions and decisions.

- Only 1 to 5% of dieters will ever achieve lasting results through dieting.

- Dieting triggers post-diet weight gain and promotes cyclical dieting.

- You can lose weight faster by eating more often and exercising less than with traditional weight-loss and dieting strategies alone.

- The truth is a hard pill to swallow.

- Knowing is the first step toward achieving the results you desire, and deserve.

- There is a better way.

2

Anatomy of a Dieter's Life

History repeats itself, but in such cunning disguise that
we never detect the resemblance until the damage is done.

– Sidney J. Harris

I can't imagine anyone starting their first diet does so believing that they are about to enter a self-perpetuating cycle of weight loss, weight gain, and dieting that can last a lifetime. But the truth is that this happens all the time, regardless of what weight loss, or dieting strategy you employ. We don't expect this could happen because we've been taught to think diets are supposed to help us lose weight and get a bit healthier. However...

If you were to examine the lives of the countless numbers of people who have employed the various weight-loss, and dieting strategies that have been available to them over the past few decades, you would find remarkable similarities in what these people experienced as a result of those weight-loss efforts – and what you're experiencing today.

Despite the shiny new wrappers, catchy names, jingles, slogans, and high-priced celebrity endorsements, the approach of modern-day weight-loss, and dieting methods is little different from what your grandparents did to lose weight twenty, thirty, even fifty years ago. And it all begins on that day when you look in the mirror and wonder... What happened?

You knew you were gaining a little weight because your clothes were getting a bit snug, but as you stare at your reflection in the mirror, you know you have to do something to get rid of the excess rolls of flesh hanging over your waistline.

Thinking you can easily do this on your own, you cut back on the treats and late-night snacks, and maybe switch to artificially sweetened or lo-cal beverages. You use 2% milk in your coffee for a while. But as time passes, the expansive nature of your waistline tells you those measures just didn't help as much as you'd have liked, so you up your game and do what you have been taught you are supposed to do when you want to lose weight: you decide to go on a diet.

You consider using one of the many plans and strategies you've heard about from friends, family, co-workers, or on the radio or television, but you also want to check what else is out there first, so you pull out your phone or tablet, or you grab your laptop, and you start searching for the latest and greatest weight-loss products, plans, and strategies available.

Your web search pulls up a seemingly unlimited stream of information, as well as advertisements about the different strategies and products available to you. And if you're lucky, you might make it through the first page or two before it all starts to blur.

After a few minutes, you decide to check out some social media sites linked to well-known weight-loss and dieting plans, and trending diet products to see what people are saying about them. And not surprisingly, you find post after post from happy dieters who have recently lost weight while using a particular plan, product, or program.

You're impressed with the endorsements offered by happy users, but you're not thrilled with the cost of some of these programs and products, so you keep your options open. Decisions, decisions… Which one will you choose? They all sound good. Hey, this one's offering a free this, and the other one is offering a free that. I can get a free month if I sign up for this one. All I have to do is pay for the food. Hmmm, how long is this going to take?

Wait? This product says it can melt away fat! Oh… when it's combined with a healthy diet and exercise. Maybe I should try this other product? It says it can boost my metabolism. Maybe I won't have to exercise so much, or give up any of my favorite foods, and its only $49 plus shipping per month for the six-month plan. Hmmm… six months is a long time. Oh…

this one also states; when combined with a healthy diet and exercise. What should I do? There's so many products and plans, how do I know what works and what doesn't?

Whether you're beginning your first diet or your twenty-first, navigating the increasing numbers of weight-loss products, plans, and programs promising to help you perfect yourself can be daunting. So, it's only natural to reach out for advice from the weight-loss experts in your life. They are the friends, family members, and co-workers who have had some success using a particular plan, product, or strategy.

Your weight-loss confidante enthusiastically agrees to share the details of his or her weight-loss success with you. They tell you of the plan, product, or strategy that has helped them to lose weight, not once or twice but three or more times, and which ones they're thinking about using the next time he or she has to lose weight. What???

You disregard the observation that your confidante has just triggered: He or she found the need to use the same or similar strategy three or more times! Maybe it's because you believe this to be the normal course of things, having grown accustomed to seeing those in your life cycle through periods of weight gain and dieting. Or, maybe it's because your confidante's plan has helped them on multiple occasions; it might be a good thing, because it might just help you, as well.

Eventually you make your decision and begin your diet, which not surprisingly starts with restricting your caloric intake and avoiding the foods everyone knows are responsible for adding unwanted pounds and inches – which are pretty much all the foods you happen to enjoy. You follow the plan to the letter, and as expected, you lose some weight. And it only took a few weeks, or months depending on how much weight you wanted to lose. Hurray You Did It!

Naturally, you're thrilled with your results. You look great, and you can't wait to share your success with the world. You eagerly tell all that inquire about how this "Amazing Weight-Loss Plan" helped you shed those unwanted pounds and inches – and maybe you even decide to share some happy pics with friends, or post them on social media. You're proud of your accomplishment, and rightfully so. What a great diet.

As time passes the excitement fades, you drift back to your regular lifestyle and the routine you've followed for years. And before you know it, you're back to your pre-diet weight – and then some. But now there's another problem. You have a function to attend that is quickly approaching, and you want to look your best. So, you call upon your faithful friend – the diet that helped whisk away those pesky pounds – and you dive head first into your next attempt to lose the same weight you had lost just a few weeks or months earlier.

As the first one or two weeks come to an end, you're going strong, but you notice this time something is a little different. The weight isn't coming off as fast as it did the first time, and your energy levels are a bit lower than normal. Not rock bottom low, but enough to make you feel like you're dragging your butt by the end of the day.

Thinking it might be something YOU are doing wrong, or something you might be eating, you try cutting even more calories from your diet. You start eliminating more foods you believe might be making it harder for you to lose weight. But your results remain unchanged. The weight isn't coming off as quickly as it did the first time, and now on top of everything else, you find yourself with less and less energy at the end of the day. You're still wondering what it is that YOU might be doing wrong.

Despite the struggle, you manage to succeed in losing some or all of the weight, and you can attend the function with your head held high. This time, you're less thrilled with your results and are just so happy it's over – but the process has left you with some new questions. Why was it harder to lose the weight, and why was your energy level so low?

You look back to see if you did something different that could explain why it was harder to lose the weight, but there was nothing. You followed the plan, same as the first time; you didn't cheat; and you even cut more calories from your diet – so what was the problem? Is it you? *My friends all lost weight this way, so why am I having such a hard time?*

With no answers in sight, you once again transition back to normal life, but this time you're not going to take any chances. You decide to watch what you eat and minimize the foods you know will add to your waistline, hoping the weight will stay off. But despite your continued vigilance, you find the weight is creeping back, and eventually you are, once again, right back where you started. You wonder: *I'm eating healthy, and I'm avoiding the bad stuff, so why am I gaining weight – Again?*

Not knowing how or why you keep gaining the weight back is frustrating, to say the least, especially when you believe you're doing everything you're supposed to. But the fact remains: you are gaining weight again, and there's only one place to point the finger of blame – yourself. After all, diets help people lose weight; it can't be the diet, so it must be you.

You wonder if the problem could be genetics, age, or a slowing metabolism. Now, to make matters worse, spring and summer are just around the corner, and there's no way you can go out looking like this. You've got to lose some weight and get in shape for the summer season, so you once again pull out your trusted diet plan and prepare to battle the bulge.

You begin the next round of dieting determined it will be different this time. You know you can do better, so you cut way back on the calories right from the start, and you eliminate all the fats and carbs that you know cause weight gain. You spend days and weeks eating salads and miniscule amounts of food at mealtime, and you swear off your favorite drinks, consuming only artificially sweetened diet beverages. You see some progress, but again, things aren't moving as quickly as you'd like them to. Maybe you should up the game a bit – add a little exercise? But who has time for that? How about some supplements to boost your efforts?

You remembered seeing something during your web search about those caffeinated supplements and those energy drinks you see everywhere. You could use them to help pick up your energy levels so you won't be tired all the time. Why not add them to the mix to help fire up the ol' furnace? You can deal with the jitters for a while if you have to, at least until you reach your goal. Hey, how about adding an appetite suppressant too? It might help with the constant hunger and cravings. (Bad idea! Don't mix weight-loss supplements unless instructed to do so by your physician.)

Having made the choice to supplement your efforts with over-the-counter stimulants and/or energy drinks, you move on with your newly modified weight-loss strategy. It's not too long before you start noticing you are, in fact, a bit jittery – maybe a little more on edge than usual – but that's okay. You can handle being a bit moodier, and you can deal with the highs and lows in your energy levels for a while – as long as the weight's coming off.

As for the constant hunger and cravings, you're a pro at this now, and you're used to being hungry all the time. You can handle it. All you need to do is keep yourself occupied, doing things that don't involve food.

The days and weeks pass slowly, but you're determined to succeed. You fight the hunger and stave off your cravings until, eventually, you reach your goal. And with a renewed faith in dieting and a greater sense of self, you once more bask in the glory of your success as you prepare to enjoy all the fun, foods, and excitement the upcoming summer season can offer.

You've conquered your weight issues. You now know exactly what you have to do when you need to lose weight. All it took was weeks or months of existing in a state of controlled starvation, and dosing yourself with caffeinated supplements, energy drinks, or appetite suppressants. Hmmm, that stuff really works. Maybe this is what you needed all along. Great Diet!

With another round of dieting behind you, you slowly drift back to your normal routine. This time, it's not just that you're happy your diet is over; your friends, family, and co-workers are happy, as well. In fact, every-one is happy your diet is over; and if you're lucky, maybe someone close to you might mention why, if no one's been mentioning it all along.

As you transition back to your normal pre-diet routine, you notice there are a couple of new things you have to deal with that weren't so obvious during your first attempts at weight loss. One of the first things you may notice is that your energy level is not bouncing back as quickly as it did following your previous diet.

You might think that's because you stopped taking the caffeinated supplements, or drinking one or more energy drinks every day, and you'd be partially right. There is a strong possibility of temporary rebound effects from prolonged use of stimulants and energy-boosting products, but it's not the only reason you may be feeling tired and be low on energy.

What you don't realize is your weight-loss efforts have triggered protective mechanisms in the body to protect the very thing you've been working so hard to lose – your fat. Protecting the remaining energy reserves stored in your fat cells is a priority for the body, and to do that, it not only restricts energy expenditure in an attempt to prevent further fat loss, leaving you low on energy, but it also triggers cravings for those foods that typically add pounds and inches quickly, in an attempt to restore the fat, you have lost.

So, with another round of dieting completed, you fully transition back to your normal routine, and throw caution to the wind; you're out to enjoy the fun, food, and festivities of the summer season. But as the season moves along, you've once again gained some or all of that weight back – and maybe a few more pounds, to boot.

Looking at your social calendar, you see that you'll have a busy fall season coming up. You have a wedding, a class reunion, and let's not forget the holidays. It's time to start all over again, but starving yourself for weeks or months isn't all that appealing, so this time you decide you're going to switch things around a bit.

Since you first started dieting, you've noticed one commercial after another for weight-loss and dieting programs, and they make dieting look so easy, so fun. *They must know something I don't know.* Everyone in those commercials always looks so happy and energetic, and they all seem to have done really well for themselves. Maybe it'll work for me, too.

Convinced this will make all the difference, you elect to move on from your mostly do-it-yourself modified weight-loss strategy to one of the pre-packaged food programs you've seen advertised. You speak with a bubbly, extremely empathetic representative who "understands" your plight, de-spite the fact she may have never been overweight a day in her life, but she's seen others struggle with weight issues and knows this plan is right for you, and it's not just because her job depends on it.

Your representative enthusiastically guides you through the sign-up process, and you fork over a few hundred bucks for your first months' worth of meals and wait for your food to show up on your doorstep. How convenient is that? You don't even have to go shopping. Just pick out what you want to eat, and that's it.

Finally, the big day arrives, and you find a nice package sitting on your doorstep when you get home from work. You wonder if it matters that it's 85 degrees in the shade, and 95 in the sun, and that your food has been sitting on the step for the past four or five hours. But it'll be alright; we've all been to barbeques where the food sits out all day. It'll be fine.

The next day you dig in with the enthusiasm of a kid at Christmas. You eat your meals and snacks, and maybe even try a meal replacement bar or one of the caffeinated meal-replacement shakes. This is great! You feel full, your energy levels are okay, and the taste isn't as bad as you thought it would be.

The first three weeks fly by and you're going strong. It couldn't be easier, and you're losing weight just like the commercial says. This is great!

You go online and fork over a few hundred dollars more, and you place your order for the upcoming weeks. You continue to do this for the next couple of months, or more, until you reach your target weight – and then it's time to Celebrate! Woohoo!

Finally, something that does exactly what it says it does, and *I didn't have to starve myself*. It was well worth the $30 per pound it cost; and besides, if I were dieting on my own, I wouldn't have been able to eat normal dinners with the family either. Drinking a meal-replacement shake before the wedding or reunion was no problem… but I am looking forward to the holidays (which is code for, I'm tired of the restrictions, and can't wait to gorge myself with my holiday favorites).

Having once again reached your goal, your diet comes to an end and your focus changes from weight loss to getting reacclimated to everyday normal foods you buy at the market. But this time the transition process is a little different. There's a lot more at stake.

Maybe you have a few boxes or bags of pre-packaged foods, shakes, and bars to use as you transition back to real whole foods, but once it's gone, you're on your own. And having just spent hundreds of dollars per month for the last few months, it would be nice to maintain your results for a while instead of just renting them. But between the holiday parties and family gatherings, before you know it the weight starts coming back with a vengeance. It's only a matter of time before you are ready for the next round. Just in time for New Year's!

Unfortunately, the next round brings with it a difficult decision: Do you continue to deal with the moodiness, constant hunger, and cravings of dieting at one-third the cost, or do you pay the price of admission for another round of program dieting? Decisions, decisions!

The program worked great, you think: I just ate too much over the holidays. Maybe if I do it again, the weight will stay off this time. But we are thinking about taking that vacation this winter, and an extra thousand dollars would go a long way. Maybe I can try one of the other weight-loss products that doesn't cost so much. After all, my New Year's resolution this year is to save more money, lose weight, and travel more – but I can't do all of that at the same time, or can I? Maybe if I try…

Each of us has a different story. The path, direction, and speed of your story may unfold differently from mine or the next person's, but…

Like it or not, this is the reality of weight loss through dieting!

This has less to do with your ability to commit to losing weight and more to do with the methods employed to do so, and how the body responds to those methods. And unless you are among the 1 to 5% of dieters with the willpower to exist in life with the restrictions, compromises, and expense of dieting (which upward of 99% of dieters find unsustainable), your life will be one continuous cycle of weight loss, weight gain, and dieting.

It's hard to believe with the advancements in nutritional science over the past few decades that no one has ever put all the pieces together. Instead, those in the weight-loss industry continue to focus on finding ways to make reducing caloric intake and/or increasing energy expenditure appealing to the consumer.

Weight-loss and diet strategies stress restriction of caloric intake as the way to lose weight. Exercise, fitness, and equipment companies offer exercise facilities, online programs, videos, and equipment to help increase your energy expenditure, burn calories, and get in shape. Supplement manufacturers stock the shelves with products designed to increase metabolism, suppress appetite, or otherwise keep you satiated. Pharmaceutical companies develop and distribute medications to suppress appetite or boost the metabolism, and food companies pump out processed lo-cal, no-cal food products by the ton.

Doctors fit patients with external devices designed to compress the stomach and minimize food intake, and surgeons perform bariatric surgery to decrease the size of your stomach or insert balloons into the stomach to occupy space and minimize the amount of food you can eat at one sitting. These are all different approaches to accomplishing the same thing: *reduce caloric intake below that of energy expenditure.*

It's not that they have it all wrong; it's that they just don't have it all right!

Because if they did have it right, there would be little need for anyone to diet more than once. So, it's time to change the way you think about weight loss and dieting. It's time to take control of your weight circumstance, and put your weight-loss and stabilization struggles behind you.

Chapter Summary

- No one starting a first diet does so believing that he or she is about to enter a self-perpetuating cycle of weight loss, weight gain, and dieting that can last a lifetime.

- The approach we use to lose weight has changed little in the past 50 to 60 years.

- It gets harder to lose weight with each attempt.

- The body responds to weight loss by protecting energy reserves stored in fat, which can result in the fatigue many dieters experience.

- Once your diet comes to an end, your body will work to restore the energy reserves stored in fat which were lost while dieting.

- Using stimulants or energy drinks can cause large fluctuations in energy levels.

- Dieting, by its very nature of how it is done, will rarely provide lasting results.

- It's not that the weight-loss and diet industry has it all wrong; they just don't have it all right!

- It's time to change the way you think about weight loss and dieting, leave the crowd behind, and take control of your weight circumstance once and for all.

3

An Industry Steeped in History

If you were to examine the history of modern-day weight-loss plans and dieting, you would find what some consider to be its humble origins some three centuries ago. It was then that the first of five notable contributions that ultimately spanned two hundred years was made. And within these five contributions lay what many believe to be the foundation for what has become a sixty-six-billion-dollar industry.

At the time these contributions were made, diets were used by physicians as treatments for the care and management of symptoms associated with various health disorders, and not for the aesthetic purposes the majority of diets are used for today. However, that situation all began to change in the mid-nineteenth century, when the third contribution stimulated a shift in public interest from weight loss as a treatment for illness to weight loss for health and aesthetic purposes.

The first notable contribution was made by a morbidly obese Scottish-born English physician, George Cheyne. Cheyne's lifestyle (and marketing strategy) involved socializing in local taverns, consuming rich food and drink, which led to morbid obesity and his failing health. Seeking to improve his weight circumstance and regain his health, Cheyne self-prescribed a *meatless diet* which involved consuming only vegetables and milk, until his health was restored.[9] Upon successfully restoring his health,

Cheyne transitioned back to his former lifestyle, only moderately restricting his dietary intake, and despite his precautions, his weight climbed and his health once again began to fail – sound familiar?

Cheyne returned to his meatless diet, regained his health, and became an advocate of vegetarianism. His book *Essays of Health and Long Life* was published in 1724, and it quickly grew in popularity, giving rise to an increased interest in and awareness of the benefits of vegetarianism.

The *second notable contribution* to modern-day weight loss and dieting came from another Scottish-born English physician, John Rollo, who was a royal artillery military surgeon. He prescribed an all-meat diet for two British soldiers who were exhibiting the symptoms of diabetes. The soldiers responded favorably to Rollo's diet, the results of which he documented in his book *Observations of Two Cases of Diabetes Mellitus*, which was published in 1797. Rollo, among other things, is credited with being the first person to develop a diet for those suffering the effects of diabetes.[10]

The *third notable contribution* is considered by many to be one of the most, if not the most, important contribution to modern-day weight loss and dieting, and it was made by William Banting, an eminent royal undertaker from London, England. The Banting family directed the funerals of King George III, King George IV, Queen Victoria, and King Edward VII, to name a few clients, but despite his eminence among funeral directors, Banting would come to be best known as the man who popularized **the low-carb diet**.[11] It was Banting's contribution that is thought to have sparked a growing public interest in weight loss for both health and aesthetic reasons. The "Banting Diet" grew in popularity with the publication of his book, *A Letter on Corpulence*, in 1863, helping to secure Banting's title as "The Father of the Low-Carb Diet."

The low-carb, high-fat diet that Banting followed was recommended by William Harvey, a Soho Square, London, physician who, under the tutelage of French physiologist Claude Bernard, learned of its benefits for the care and management of those suffering with diabetes. The Banting Diet, or the "Banting Harvey Diet," as it was called, focused on minimizing consumption of starchy foods and sugars, and this sparked a growing interest in weight loss and dieting. Over 150 years later, refined versions of this Banting Diet continue to be one of the most commonly used strategies for those seeking to lose a few pounds and inches.

The *fourth notable contribution* maybe considered as both a gift and a curse for dieters. It is the calorie: the unit measure of energy we use to regulate our dietary intake. A calorie is the amount of energy it takes to heat 1 gram of water 1 degree Celsius. Capitalize the word *Calorie* and it changes the definition to this: the amount of energy it takes to heat 1 kilogram of water 1 degree Celsius (The kilocalorie). Today, the calorie is used to represent the amount of energy a serving of a particular food can provide the body.

Although there is some controversy as to who actually discovered the calorie, credit for the earliest use of the term goes to Frenchman Nicholas Clement who, as early as 1819, referred to the calorie as a unit of heat energy.[12] But the calorie, as it were, had no ties to food or nutrition until 1848, when German physician Julius Mayer opened discussions that food was a source of energy for the body. Prior to that time, the vast majority of the population believed that energy, or our ability to function, was solely a gift of divine origins.

It would take thirty-nine years from the time Mayer first suggested food was the body's source of energy before the calorie was introduced to the United States, in 1887, as a nutritional unit of measure. This was done by Wilbur Atwater, an American chemist known for his studies of human nutrition and metabolism. Atwater's work essentially laid the groundwork for modern-day nutrition.[13]

The *fifth notable contribution* came nearly two centuries after physician George Cheyne published his *Essays of Health, and Long Life*, which touted the benefits of a vegetarian diet, and is still considered by many to be the most influential and applicable contribution to modern-day weight loss and dieting. This last contribution was made by Dr. Lulu Hunt Peters, who widely popularized counting calories with her book *Diet and Health, with Key to the Calories*, published in 1918.

Peters was an American doctor. She wrote a featured column called *Diet and Health* for the Central Press Association, with distribution to four hundred newspapers having a cumulative readership of 12 million people. Dr. Peters' book sold over 2 million copies, to become the first bestselling weight-loss and dieting book in history. It remained among the top ten nonfiction books from 1922 to 1926.[14]

The book promoted something that was fairly new to the world at the time: counting calories. And it's timing couldn't have been better. The U.S. government, in response to the global food shortage caused by World War I, was seeking ways to reduce food consumption by the American population. To encourage Americans to eat less, the government issued a "Scientific Diet," and the cornerstone of this diet' was – you guessed it – counting calories. Fueled by patriotism, calorie-conscious Americans shifted toward a "the thinner, the better" mentality, and "reducing" became all the rage.[15]

'Reducing' was one of the first, if not the first, weight-loss craze in America. It had little to do with health and nutrition, and more to do with getting thin by whatever means necessary – and everyone wanted to be part of it. The "thin is in" trend was off and running, and calorie counting offered a sensible, seemingly healthy solution from a recognized authority on weight loss and dieting.

Today, counting calories is more popular than ever, and it is practiced by dieters the world over. It is considered by many to be a necessary step in the weight-loss process, but it is also how dieters get themselves into trouble. That's because few people understand the effects that restricting one's caloric intake can have on the body, and on meeting post-diet caloric needs.

As important as counting calories may be for some people, there are details associated with caloric restriction that many dieters are unaware of. It is in the details that we find those things that can interfere with weight-loss and weight-stabilization efforts. These are details that can cost you more than just your hard-earned results.

The world we live in has changed. Our food sources have changed, and so, too, must we change how we approach weight loss and stabilization.

Chapter Summary

- Modern-day weight loss and dieting can trace its origins back nearly three centuries.

- Physician George Cheyne's book *Essays of Health and Long Life* sparked a interest in and awareness of the benefits of vegetarianism in 1724.

- Physician John Rollo prescribed and an all-meat diet to soldiers suffering the effects of diabetes to help manage their symptoms, and he is credited with being the first to develop a diet specifically for those suffering the effects of diabetes. His book *Observations of Two Cases of Diabetes Mellitus* was published in 1797.

- In 1819, Frenchman Nicholas Clement first used the word *calorie* as a unit of heat energy.

- German physician Julian Mayer in 1848 opened the dialogue on food as being the body's source of energy. Prior to that, our ability to function was thought to be of divine origins.

- William Banting, a renowned royal undertaker, is credited in 1863 with popularizing the low-carb diet, known as the "Banting Diet," in his book *A Letter on Corpulence*. Banting is considered to be "The Father of the Low Carb Diets," an idea still in use today, 150 years later.

- In 1887, American chemist Wilbur Atwater introduced the calorie to the United States as a measure of nutritional value.

- Dr. Lulu Hunt Peters popularized counting calories in 1918, with her bestselling book *Diet and Health, With Key to the Calories*.

- Today, counting calories is more popular than ever, and it is one way most dieters get themselves into trouble.

4

Dieting Pitfalls

*Sometimes, looking back is exactly
what we need to move us forward.*

– Unknown

When I discovered the truth about weight loss and dieting, it immediately brought to mind a memory from my childhood. I remembered a group of women from the neighborhood who all started to use the latest and greatest weight-loss and dieting strategy of the time. Even as a young boy with no interest in the topic, I couldn't help but know what they were doing, because it was all they talked about, whether at home, on the phone, or at neighborhood social gatherings. But there was one person among them I remember most.

It was the daughter of one of my neighbors, about a year or so younger than I was. She was the youngest of three children in her family. I remember her as a sweet kid, not timid, but far less outgoing than her older sister and her brother. She wasn't sickly, and certainly she wasn't obese as a young child. In fact, I can't remember her looking anything more than a little overweight – before she started dieting.

As kids go, she wasn't very active, and for whatever reason, she rarely joined in the games and other activities the neighborhood kids played.

While we were running around, playing ball, tag, or riding our bicycles, she was inside the house, and when she did come outside, she would usually sit on the steps in front of her home and watch the rest of us playing.

What I remember most about her, though, were her sudden dramatic mood and weight swings. Her mother had put her on the same weight-loss plan that the other neighborhood women were using, which I can only imagine had to be extremely difficult for a young girl. While every other kid in the neighborhood was eating what they wanted at neighborhood barbeques, parties, and gatherings, or were chasing the ice cream truck, her mother – with good intentions, I'm sure – would govern what she could and couldn't eat, based upon the recommendations of this miracle diet that all the adults were following, off and on, over a few years.

Avoiding your favorite foods is difficult enough for adults. Now, imagine taking your kids' favorite foods away from them. The same foods you as a parent allowed them to eat freely, but now are taking away and expecting them to understand why they have to restrict what they eat while every other kid in the neighborhood gets to eat what he or she wants, including those kids who are heavier.

Often, I would see her at these gatherings, and her mother would be arguing with her about something she wanted to eat but couldn't because it wasn't on the plan. On more than one occasion, she ended up leaving the gathering and not returning. In fact, I'd watch as each of them, women and men alike cycled through periods of weight loss, weight gain, and dieting, all to lose the same weight again and again. And even at that age, I found it strange that anyone would repeatedly pay to lose the same weight. Little did I know the profound affect this memory would have when later, as an adult it dawned on me, I had just gone through five years of doing the exact same thing – the same thing I watched that girl, her mother, and a number of women, and men from the neighborhood go through thirty years earlier. To my mind, nothing in weight loss had changed.

Sadly, my neighbor's weight circumstance did not improve as she grew up. The most vivid memory I have of her was seeing her in the driveway of her parent's home, wearing a muumuu house dress that was more fitting for an elderly, obese relative than for a young girl in her early to mid-teens.

So, I turned my focus to the one thing we had in common: dieting. I was determined to find out if there was something about dieting that might be responsible for the struggles not only of my childhood neighbors but also of upwards of 99% of dieters today. And it wasn't long before I found what I was looking for.

I noticed a number of pitfalls common to the most popular weight-loss and dieting strategies:

- Restriction
- Sustainability
- Transitioning
- Stabilization

Each of these factors is an essential part of the dieting process, and each plays a crucial role in your ability to achieve the lasting results you desire, and deserve. It is only by understanding each factor, and how it can work for or against your weight-loss and weight-stabilization efforts, that you can turn the tide in your favor.

Restriction

The cornerstone of most weight-loss and dieting strategies is the restriction of caloric intake below that of energy expenditure. And there is no question that this approach is necessary for anyone who wishes to shed unwanted pounds and inches. However, restricting your caloric intake is a double-edged sword. It is both hero and villain.

When we restrict caloric intake, and the body begins to release fat, the circulating levels of an appetite-controlling hormone called *leptin* begin to decrease. Leptin's job is to maintain your body weight within a fairly narrow range, regardless of your starting weight, and it does this by controlling appetite and energy expenditure.

When the body detects a decrease in circulating levels of leptin, it interprets this as a loss in the energy reserves stored in fat, and so it responds by trying to conserve the body's remaining energy reserves. One way it does this is by restricting the amount of energy being used for non-vital functions.

If you have ever wondered why you get cold when you're dieting, this is it. One of the things your body does to prevent excess energy expenditure is to limit the amount of energy used in maintaining body temperature. It does this is by shifting blood away from your extremities and directing it toward your body's core.

Another way the body works to protect its stored energy reserves is by slowing the metabolism. When dieters talk about metabolism, they are actually talking the body's metabolic rate, or the amount of time it takes to process and burn the calories we get from the foods we consume. But metabolism is much more than our ability to burn calories.

Metabolism is the sum total of all biochemical reactions of the mind and body needed for the body to function and survive. In weight loss, this includes all the physical and chemical processes that convert the proteins, fats, and carbohydrates we consume into the energy and essential nutrients the body uses for cell growth, repair, maintenance, and function. But conserving energy and protecting the remaining fat stores is only the first step. The body also responds to lower levels of Leptin by cranking up the dial on your appetite – which for dieters means cravings.

Here's the problem. Leptin is made and released by your fat cells. The more fat you lose, the lower your leptin levels get. So, every time you try and crank up the furnace on your fat-burning machine, your body works hard to shut it down, which in part accounts for the slow progress many dieters make in their efforts to shed those unwanted pounds.

Where dieters get into trouble when restricting their caloric intake is that they *believe* less is better. But as evidence suggests, this has not been the case for the majority of dieters. It may seem like a good idea to skip meals or to eat scant amounts of food on and off throughout the day, so as to take the edge off the constant hunger most dieters experience when dieting, but eating this way, or not eating at all, can contribute to slowing your metabolism even more.

As a dieter, you might see the problem this causes. Your goal is to lose weight and release unwanted accumulations of fat clinging to various parts of your body, but the hormone leptin is made by the body's fat cells, and when you restrict your caloric intake and begin to release fat, your leptin levels decrease as well – triggering the body's response to prevent further depletion of energy reserves stored in your fat cells while at the same time stimulating your appetite in an attempt to rebuild those fat stores.

This makes your weight-loss efforts increasingly difficult when you are unware of how to counter the effects that restricted caloric intake has on the body. This means restriction is the first pitfall that dieters must learn to address if they wish to improve the results of their weight-loss efforts.

Sustainability

One of the most challenging aspects of weight loss and dieting is the ability to sustain your weight-loss efforts long enough to achieve your goal or target weight. Let's face it; dieting the way we have been shown to do it is a struggle. We force ourselves to make radical dietary changes that affect almost every aspect of our lives, and expect to maintain our efforts for extended periods of time.

It's no wonder the majority of dieters fail to achieve the desired results. But it's not just the dietary changes, restrictions, and compromises we make when dieting that turns weight loss into a struggle. There are other factors equally responsible for bringing our weight-loss efforts to an end. Together, they make sustainability the second pitfall of dieting that needs to be addressed if you wish to achieve lasting results.

The ability to sustain your weight-loss efforts has less to do with your desire or commitment to lose weight, and more to do with the approach you use to do so. Most diets not only restrict caloric intake, they also alter your dietary intake by removing the foods you have come to enjoy eating.

Researchers believe that some of the foods we consume have an addictive quality, and when ingested, they trigger the release of endorphins. These are the body's feel-good chemicals, which makes eliminating them from your dietary intake even more difficult.

The foods we consume provide us a certain amount of comfort, and when we try to remove those foods from our lives for extended periods of time, without replacing them with something equally satisfying, tasty, and comforting, we add to those factors that make traditional weight-loss and dieting strategies unsustainable.

The methods we employ to lose weight vary with age and intent. On one end of the weight-loss spectrum, there are vanity dieters. They are those people who are always on a diet. They watch every morsel of food that goes into their mouths, and they exercise daily. They are motivated by appearance, and they continually strive to perfect themselves, so their weight-loss and stabilization efforts tend to be more of an obsession.

On the other end of the spectrum are those who diet out of medical necessity. They have either been prescribed a specific diet to help manage medical conditions like diabetes, heart disease, bowel disorders, food allergies, and intolerances, or for whatever reasons have become so obese that medical intervention is necessary to preserve their lives. And although their numbers remain relatively low, the numbers of those suffering with extreme obesity are on the rise.

The majority of us fall between the two ends of the spectrum, and we simply want to improve our appearance, get a bit healthier, and maybe feel a little better about ourselves. We are those who wish to improve our health and the quality of life. We are the masses without the time or desire to incorporate lengthy radical dietary changes, or aggressive exercise regimens, into already hectic lifestyles. We are just seeking a better way to improve the effects that time and lifestyle have had on our bodies.

Eighty percent of dieters are do-it-yourselfers, and they employ traditional methods of restricting caloric intake in attempts to release unwanted pounds and inches. They cut back on carbs, fats, and sugars, and eliminate those foods they have been led to believe are responsible for their weight circumstance.

Some will try to incorporate less regimented forms of exercise in an attempt to tone up, and others will seek the help of the latest and greatest weight-loss potions, pills, and products whipped up by modern-day alchemists in an attempt to regain their former figures. The remaining 20% will stand cash in hand, ready to pay the price of admission for another attempt to lose the same weight they lost only a few weeks or months earlier.

Each strategy provides results, but what it all boils down to is your being able to stick to the plan or strategy you've selected long enough to achieve your goals – which for the majority of dieters has proven itself to be one of the most difficult aspects of dieting.

The average dieter will lose approximately 4 to 6 pounds during the first week of dieting, but as most dieters are aware, this does not mean you've lost 4 to 6 pounds of fat. The majority of weight released during the first week of dieting comes from the elimination of water. We'll get more into that a little later on.

In the weeks to follow, the average dieter can expect to lose 1 to 2 pounds per week following the most commonly used weight-loss and dieting strategies. So, if you want to lose 10 pounds, you can expect to accomplish this in as few as three to four weeks, or as many as six or seven weeks, depending on your physical health and other factors influencing your weight-loss efforts.

Now let's push that goal of losing 10 pounds up to 20, and it will take anywhere from eight to sixteen weeks or more to shed those unwanted pounds and inches. A goal of 30 pounds can set you back three to six months, or more. At 40 pounds, odds are another birthday will pass before you can hope to hit your target weight.

The math is easy enough, but this is where dieters run into trouble. Recent studies suggest that the average diet will only last five weeks, two days, and forty-three minutes.[16] Now, that's pretty specific, but according to a UK research study involving 1,000 women, the average length of time before willpower gave in to the constant hunger and relentless cravings of dieting was less than six weeks – which means that if you're looking to lose more than 10 to 15 pounds, you're pretty much up that creek without a paddle.

One of the reasons the majority of diets come to an end within the first six weeks is that there are a number of factors to which dieters remain unaware, which influence weight-loss efforts. There are the physical, emotional, social, and financial factors that can end your weight-loss efforts as quickly as they began.

For example, younger dieters tend to be more prone to the emotional, social, and financial pressures of dieting, and have a tendency to give up quickly on their weight-loss efforts. Many do so within the first few weeks. Younger dieters also tend to diet more frequently than their older counterparts who appear less susceptible to the emotional, social, and financial pressures of dieting affording them the potential to sustain their weight loss efforts a bit longer lengthening the cycle of weight loss, weight gain and dieting to lose the same weight repeatedly. But only marginally.

We also need to consider time as the enemy. The longer you diet, the more time those factors influencing sustainability have to work against your weight-loss efforts when you don't know how to address them. And how can you address something you aren't aware even exists?

Indeed, the factors interfering with your ability to sustain your weight-loss efforts are not limited to your ability to restrict caloric intake. There are physical adaptation issues, or plateaus, that dieters reach where weight-loss efforts produce little or no results.[17] Additionally, there are psychological factors, emotional matters, and environmental issues that play an equally important role in the ability to stay the course.

Have you ever considered the effects that dieting has on your social life? Few dieters do, until they're experiencing them. Instinctively, we want to be part of something bigger than ourselves (no pun intended). It's part of human nature to want to fit in, to belong, which is why many of us go on a diet to begin with – to fit in. To look the same or better than those around us. That's why we seek safety, and comfort in numbers, with family and friends. It's a herding mentality that, much like the *fight or flight instinct*, developed as a result of learned experience that has been passed down through countless generations over the millennia, and have become part of the body's operating system.

But when we diet, we separate ourselves from family and friends at meal time. You may be sitting with family and friends, but inside you know you're sitting at the table eating a meal-replacement bar, drinking a shake, or eating another salad with a dry piece of grilled chicken on top – while everyone else is enjoying the foods you have eliminated from your diet. This not only tests your willpower, it also adds to the stress and anxiety of dieting.

This may be one of the reasons why some weight-loss strategies offer a "cheat day" during the week, which in theory is a good way to help put your cravings at bay for a while, provided you don't go overboard and wipe out the results achieved in the prior days and weeks. This strategy also helps you connect socially with friends and family at mealtime without restriction at least once per week, which may help in the social aspects of sustainability.

Sustainability issues affect every dieter, do-it-yourselfer, and program dieter. Increasing numbers of diet plans promote the consumption of everything from whole foods with personal support, and instruction, to prepackaged foods delivered by mail, which seems a convenient option. But these, too, present with their own sustainability issues. They come with a cost, which many cannot afford.

The average do-it yourself (DIY) dieter can easily spend well over $100 per month on diet foods, products, supplements, and beverages. Program dieters can spend in excess of $300 or more per month by the time they finish buying all the food, extras, and support. Both approaches help you lose unwanted pounds and inches as long as you follow the plan, but what happens when you can no longer foot the bill?

It's here that many dieters hit the financial wall. That space between desire and end goal is just too wide and too costly to sustain. Paying an extra $300 per month to lose an average of 8 to 10 pounds per month is not an option for everyone, and an extra $100 or more spent on top of your monthly grocery bill can go a long way toward helping with other, more important expenses, or that family vacation you wanted to take, expanding your wardrobe, or upgrading to that new car you've always wanted.

In sum, if you cannot do what you are doing to lose weight, whether physically, emotionally, or financially, your weight-loss efforts will come to an end. Learning to address these issues is essential to both your short- and long-term weight-loss success; in most cases, can be easily accomplished with nothing more than delicious real foods you can pick up at any market, and can prepare and share with family and friends.

Transitioning

The next point marks both the happiest stage of your weight-loss efforts and what can be the most frustrating time for experienced dieters. It is the day your diet comes to an end and you begin to transition back to life as you knew it before dieting.

It's a happy day if you've succeeded in reaching your weight-loss goals, and now you can rejoin life as you knew it before your diet began. But as any experienced dieter knows, it's also the day when the results achieved through weeks and months of effort start to reverse themselves.

Post-diet weight gain is part and parcel of every calorie-restrictive weight-loss and dieting strategy because, while your weight-loss efforts have come to an end, your body will continue to do what it is programmed to do: restore lost energy reserves stored in fat. Once your diet comes to an end, the body can work to rebuild those lost fat reserves, now unchecked by dietary restrictions. This means weight gain.

When you begin to add calories back into your dietary intake, you do so with a slower metabolism. You may think you're eating healthy, and you might be for someone who hasn't just come off weeks of dieting, but the fact is that your body has accommodated to that reduced caloric intake and will now take full advantage of the opportunity to restore what was lost.

As a dieter, you are likely aware of the general guidelines for the recommended number of calories per day you need to consume to maintain your weight and normal bodily functions, but did you know that the actual number of calories your body requires varies depending on a number of factors, weight loss included. If you try to stick to that rule after your diet has come to an end, you may find yourself shopping for larger clothes sooner rather than later.

General daily caloric intake guidelines vary by source.

Age	Sedentary Women	Sedentary Men	Active Women	Active Men
18-30 years	2000 calories/day	2400 calories/day	2400 calories/day	3000 calories/day
31-50 years	1800 calories/day	2200 calories/day	2200 calories/day	2800 calories/day
51+ years	1600 calories/day	2000 calories/day	2000 calories/day	2600 calories/day

Let's say you just spent the last ten to twelve weeks losing the 20 pounds you gained sitting behind the desk at your new job, and you begin to transition back to your normal lifestyle. You know the rule: you're 28 years old and not very active in your new position. You believe if you keep your caloric intake at or below 2000/2400 calories per day, you will maintain your post-diet weight. But over time, you realize you're gaining weight despite following those guidelines. You can't help but wonder. Why?

What you may not be aware of is that the body's metabolism can slow by as much as 24% over the course of the twelve weeks of dieting.[18] And when you begin to add more calories to your daily intake, doing so with a slower metabolism, you allow your body to restore the lost fat reserves.

Your body has adapted to the change in your caloric intake, and the number of calories you now need to maintain and stabilize your weight has also decreased.[19] This means that when you return to eating a well-balanced diet based on that recommended number of calories for someone of your age, sex and activity level, you are actually consuming too many calories for what is now normal for your body. The result? Weight gain!

Unfortunately, there is little helpful information available about the proper way to transition to your normal routine. That may be because no matter how you transition back, post-diet weight gain is inevitable. Maybe that's why no one in the weight-loss industry has offered much in the way of transitioning advice. As it is right now, dieters hold their weight-loss strategies and programs in the highest regard. After all, they help us to lose weight, and we believe that any post-diet weight gain is of our own doing.

Now, if that's your thinking, you have no other place than yourself to point the finger of blame, otherwise your perception of weight loss and dieting would be negatively affected, and we wouldn't want that now, would we?

The key to minimizing the effects of transitioning, or of eliminating them altogether, is to gradually transition to real foods as your diet comes to an end. In doing so, your body can accommodate the increase in caloric intake slowly, minimizing the effects. Gradual transitioning combined with an effective and sustainable maintenance plan will help you maintain more of the results of your weight-loss efforts indefinitely.

Maintenance and Stabilization

The final factor in weight loss and dieting is maintenance. Much like transitioning, there is a remarkable lack of information available about how to stabilize and maintain your new weight and waistline once your diet comes to an end. One might venture to guess that this is by design, but that would be an unfair assessment of the weight-loss industry and the programs available.

Many dieters seem to harbor the misconception that once their diet comes to an end, the weight should stay off as long as they watch what they eat. But as any seasoned dieter can tell you, this is not the reality. Eventually, we drift back to our old ways, and sooner or later we find the need to once again go on a diet.

Most diet plans offer little to no information on maintenance, not by design, act, or omission but, rather, because their goal is to help you lose weight, and maintain your results by changing your dietary habits to their version of a healthy diet. Unfortunately, admirable intentions often prove to be too drastic and too difficult a change to comfortably incorporate into our lives indefinitely.

The majority of dieters have little or no desire to completely change their dietary habits. They're just looking for a better way to manage their weight, and maybe get a bit healthier in the process. They want to continue enjoying their favorite foods. Most people, myself included, find dramatic lifestyle changes, whether dietary or otherwise, difficult to accomplish and maintain for extended periods of time.

Further, radical dietary changes are hard enough to incorporate into your life when you live on your own, but when you have a partner and/or other family members who have no need or desire to accommodate these changes, that adds stress to your weight-loss and stabilization efforts.

Transitioning and maintenance are key to lasting results, and can be accomplished simply by knowing how your body responds to weight loss, dieting, and the foods you consume. In knowing this, you can transition gradually, slowly lifting the restrictions and the compromises associated with dieting, and can ease your way into a lifestyle that allows you to enjoy all foods sensibly, with friends and family, without having to worry about permanent weight gain.

It is the process of learning how to eat and grow thin that will give you the ability to manage your weight and waistline with an accuracy unlike you've ever known before. When you understand how your body responds to your weight-loss efforts, and how the foods and combinations of foods you consume can work for or against your weight loss and stabilization efforts, you will hold the keys to success. It may sound too good to be true now, but it's easier than you may think.

Once you learn how to address the pitfalls of dieting and the barriers to success, and acknowledge the changes that go unaddressed by today's weight-loss and dieting strategies, you will have the knowledge and tools to stabilize a healthier weight and waistline.

Learn this, and you will have what has eluded dieters for the better part of a century:

Control!

Chapter Summary

- The results dieters experience today is little different from those experienced by dieters' decades ago.

- Restriction, sustainability, transitioning, and maintenance are the four primary factors inherent in most common weight-loss and dieting strategies in use today.

- Weight loss, and decreasing levels of leptin, triggers a physiological response in the body to minimize the loss of energy stored in fat, making your weight-loss efforts increasingly difficult.

- Leptin is made by the fat cells.

- The body conserves energy by minimizing the energy used to heat the body, and by slowing the metabolism.

- Metabolism is the sum total of all physical and chemical reactions in the body necessary to maintain life and normal function.

- Metabolic rate is the speed at which we burn the calories from the foods we consume.

- Sustainability in weight loss and dieting is the ability to physically, emotionally, or financially continue your chosen weight-loss strategy until you reach your goal or target weight.

- Transitioning from dieting to normal routine is the point where the hard-earned results achieved through your weight-loss efforts begin to reverse themselves.

- Transitioning and Maintenance is the key to achieving lasting results, and can be done with little compromise while enjoying all foods sensibly.

- Learning to address the pitfalls inherent in dieting, and the barriers, blocks, and changes interfering with your weight management efforts, will give you what has eluded dieters for the better part of a century – control!

5

The AHA Moment

AHA moments are funny things. You can be racking your brain for hours, days, weeks, and even months trying to figure something out, and nothing happens. You just can't find the answers you are looking for, no matter how hard you try. Then you hop in your car, and a good song comes on the radio, or you walk into another room and see something on the television, and Bam! The answer pops into your head, and you can't help but think; *It was so obvious... why didn't I see it before?*

It could be anything that triggers your inspiration, and more times than not, it's something that has absolutely nothing to do with the problem at hand. It's almost as if it were a lesson, telling us that sometimes we need to step back from the problem, let it go for a while, and then look at it with a fresh perspective.

An AHA moment, as defined by Webster, is "a moment of sudden realization, inspiration, insight, recognition, or comprehension." It is the moment when lightning strikes, and the solution you've been looking for, or the path you need to take, appears right in front of you.

It was shortly after finishing the last in a string of diets I had begun five-years earlier in an attempt to lose the 10 pounds gained after my injury and surgery that the lightning struck. I was sitting in front of my computer, thinking about why I couldn't stabilize my weight after my many diets had come to an end, when I looked down at my glasses, and BAM! It hit me.

Weight gain is not the problem... It's a symptom!

Ever since Dr. Lulu Hunt Peters popularized counting calories in 1918 with her book *Diet & Health: With Key to the Calories,* the weight-loss and diet industry has focused solely on the reduction of caloric intake in one form or another to help those in need lose weight. But what if there is something else other than overeating that also causes us to gain weight? And what if it interfered with our ability to lose weight – and keep it off as well?

Find that something, and it would be like finding the missing piece of the weight-loss puzzle. Learn how to address it, and it would be the key to improving the effectiveness of any weight-loss effort. It would provide a means to stabilize and maintain a healthier weight and waistline indefinitely. It would, in essence, be a cure for dieting.

I was reminded that from the moment we are born to the moment we die; our bodies are in a constant state of change. From birth through our early twenties, we are growing and developing; beyond that, it's all about maintaining the cells, tissues, and organs, and preserving functionality. But as efficient as the body may be at maintaining itself, it's only natural for the organs, tissues, and cells to degrade and decrease in efficiency over time. It's called aging. But time alone does not dictate the aging process or the efficiency of systemic functions.

Aging is a genetically determined process. It is a progressive deterioration of physiological function.[20] It is the effect that time has on the body, which can be dramatically influenced and accelerated by lifestyle, dietary choices, and environmental factors.

Some of the changes affecting our bodies over time are obvious. When our vision begins to blur, we know to get glasses, or contacts, or have laser surgery to correct the problem. If our hair is thinning, graying, or worse, we use hair-growth products or have hair-replacement procedures to address the issue. When and if our hearing starts to decline, we get hearing aids to improve our hearing, and if we develop joint pain, we get braces to support the affected joints, or we exercise, get therapy, or have surgery to correct the problem.

These are all obvious bodily changes we either see, feel, or otherwise notice, and we can address the cause of it as needed. We accept these changes as a normal part of life, whether the result of lifestyle, aging, genetics, or the wear and tear of living. But other changes occurring in the body are not so obvious.

These changes are what is referred to by the healthcare community as "subclinical," or the changes that occur in the body that are not severe enough to present definite or readily observable symptoms. But it's often what we don't see that gives us the most trouble.

It would be absurd to think that just because we can't see or feel something that it does not change along with everything else. Every year millions of people are diagnosed with health-related issues that have been developing for years, yet they never knew that because those issues weren't obvious enough to be addressed. They couldn't see or feel what was happening until things got bad enough to be symptomatic. But not being severe enough to cause symptoms does not mean these changes do not affect the efficiency of bodily functions.

Cavities don't just appear overnight. It can take months, or even years, for those cavities to develop.[21] You won't know you have a cavity until the decay from acids and bacteria in your mouth have eroded the enamel enough to expose the sensitive tissue it protects. You didn't see it happening, but none the less it was happening.

Kidney stones, gallstones, benign prostatic hypertrophy, osteopenia, osteoporosis, fatty liver, glaucoma, insulin resistance, leptin resistance, osteoarthritis, and carpal tunnel syndrome are all examples of changes affecting different parts of the body, and all of them are influenced by genetics, lifestyle, and/or dietary choices. Each can take years to develop, and each affects the function of the organ or system it is associated with.

Lightning often strikes when we least expect it.

Everything has a cause, and where there is a cause, there is a remedy.

How many people are living with varying degrees of cardiovascular disease and don't know it because they can't see or feel what's happening inside themselves. It is estimated that 85.6 million Americans are living with some form of cardiovascular disease.[22] The majority of these people have no idea because the changes are not yet obvious, but that doesn't mean the function of their heart is not in one way or another affected by these changes.

Of these people, the ones who are fortunate will experience mild symptoms as the condition progresses, like lightheadedness, labored breathing with minimal exertion, fatigue, or dizziness. Those conditions can alert us that something is wrong, and we need to get checked out. Sadly, for some, the first sign that something is wrong is the last sign.

According the American Heart Association, cardiovascular disease is the leading cause of premature death.[23] One in four deaths in the United States is directly related to overweight and obesity – over 650,000 per year.[24] Overweight and obesity is the fifth leading risk for global deaths. At least 2.8 million adults die each year as a result of being overweight or obese.[25]

What's interesting is that the Centers for Disease Control (CDC) documents the annual number of deaths related to overweight and obesity, but it doesn't list obesity as a cause of death. Instead, it lists heart disease as the no. 1 cause of death, which suggests that overweight and obesity are so closely linked to heart disease that they are reported as one and the same thing for one in four people who die each year as a direct or indirect result of being overweight.

The point is that for the most part, we remain unaware of the less obvious or subclinical changes affecting our bodies. It is only when those changes have progressed far enough along to become symptomatic that we seek to address them. Which in some cases is too late.

It would be foolish to think that the digestive system does not degrade in function over time, or that genetics, lifestyle, dietary choices, and environmental factors do not influence the efficiency of the GI system as well. So, how does this relate to weight gain, as well as our ability to stabilize and maintain a healthy weight and waistline?

The body's ability to efficiently process and assimilate the foods we consume degrades overtime, along with every other system in the body. These changes occur naturally with age, but the rapid increase in childhood obesity strongly suggests that the process is accelerated not only by dietary factors, but by physical, genetic, and environmental factors as well.

Overweight and obesity have reached epidemic proportions. The CDC estimates that 75% or more of the U.S. population will be overweight or obese by the year 2020.[26] It is increasingly apparent that dieting on its own is not helping to reduce the growing numbers of overweight and obese people. In fact, according to medical and nutritional research, dieting is contributing to the overweight and obesity epidemic.[27]

It was in this one moment, my aha moment, that I saw the course I needed to follow. The task I committed myself to was finding that which goes unaddressed by the weight-loss and dieting industry and as employed by dieters the world over.

We all know overeating leads to overweight and obesity, but what causes overeating? There is no lack of information on the emotional and psychological reasons why some people overeat, but the majority of dieters are not afflicted with such long-term emotional eating disorders. Nor do they eat excessive amounts of junk foods, fast foods, or sweets on a regular basis.

Of course, it's only natural that we have a bad day once in a while, and maybe on those occasions we seek the comfort of a favorite food or we overindulge in something we know we shouldn't have. But that's not every day or every week, and the occasional overindulgence should not dramatically affect our weight.

We are creatures of habit. Most of us have been eating and drinking the same foods and beverages in the same quantities our entire life, and we are just is active as we've always been. We have maintained our weight, give or take a few pounds, over the years. Then out of the blue, it's as if someone threw a switch. Bam! We start gaining weight. The phrase coined for this insidious change is "middle age spread," or MAS.

MAS is defined as an increase in bulk, especially in the waist, buttocks, and hips, traditionally associated with the onset of middle age and the body's decreasing ability to metabolize calories efficiently.[28] This definition provides the smoking gun.

The "middle age" in MAS traditionally was reserved for those in their late twenties, thirties, and forties, and the" spread" part was a result of decreased core strength, muscle tone, and a decrease in the body's ability to process and assimilate the foods we consume into fat-burning energy. Unfortunately, this is no longer the case. MAS has evolved to include an increasing number of younger people as well. It's not uncommon for people in their early to mid-twenties (and younger) to experience "early onset middle age spread," or EAS.

The question I had was: Why? What are those things in life, in our bodies, and in the environment that are responsible for accelerating the process of degradation that in the recent past was reserved for much older individuals, but now affects adults who are young and old, as well as the rapidly growing numbers of overweight children?

It wasn't long before I discovered a number of factors common to each of us that contribute to overweight and obesity. They are the barriers, blocks, and changes we'll be looking at next.

Chapter Summary

- Aha moments are moments of sudden realization, inspiration, insight, recognition, or comprehension. It is the moment when lightning strikes.

- Weight gain is not the problem; it's a symptom!

- Age is a genetically determined process, but we don't have to help it along.

- Over 650,000 deaths each year are a direct result of overweight and obesity.

- 85.6 million people are walking around with some degree of heart disease and don't even know it.

- The CDC estimates upwards of 75% of the U.S. population will be overweight or obese by 2020.

- Dieting is contributing to the overweight and obesity epidemic by triggering post-diet weight gain.

- Cyclical dieting comes with a cost far beyond the monetary expense.

- Middle age spread is the result of decreased core strength, increased adiposity, decreased levels of physical activity, and decrease in digestive efficiency.

- Middle age spread has evolved to include an increasing number of young adults.

6

The Barriers, Blocks, and Changes

Having realized that weight gain is a symptom, and not the problem, was a game changer for me. This meant looking at weight loss from an entirely different perspective, and as all symptoms have causes, I began examining the reasons why we gain weight and why upwards of 99% of dieters' struggle with weight loss and fail to maintain a healthier weight and waistline.

At first, I focused on the physical aspects of weight gain. Then, one after another, the barriers, blocks, and changes influencing our ability to efficiently manage our weight began to line up. I call them the BBCs. They are the physical, genetic, environmental, and psychological factors that control weight-loss efforts and that dictate our weight circumstance. They support weight gain, impede the progress of weight-loss efforts, and interfere with the ability to stabilize and maintain the hard-earned results of weight-loss efforts.

If we learn to address the BBCs, we will have the key to unlock the secret, and experience an efficiency unlike any we've known before. Each of these barriers, blocks, and changes on its own is capable of influencing the waistline and your weight-loss efforts, but truth be told, most dieters have all or some of them to contend with.

If it is the truth you seek, you will often find it
buried under a mound of misinformation and misdirection.
Truth is not always kind, but at least it is honest.

I began to understand why no one, to the best of my knowledge, has ever done anything to address the cumulative role that these barriers, blocks, and changes play in our weight-loss efforts. But times are changing, and with the growing overweight and obesity epidemic, it has become ever more important to understand the bigger picture.

The Physical Barriers

The physical barriers have little to do with your physical strength, or your ability to strengthen yourself with a regimented exercise program, and more to do with the effects that time, age, dieting, diet, and exposure to the increasing amounts of chemicals, pollutants, and toxins have on the body's ability to efficiently process, and assimilate the foods we consume.

The digestive system is one of the most efficient processing plants on the planet. It not only takes in raw materials in the form of the foods we consume, and breaks them down through the process of digestion into the essential nutrients, and energy the body requires to maintain normal bodily functions. It is also the cornerstone of your immune system. The digestive system is the front line in protecting us from harmful bacteria, pathogens, and parasites that enter the body, and is estimated to make up 80% of the body's immune response.[29]

The physical barriers include both internal, and external factors which contribute to your weight circumstance. On the surface, some of these seem harmless enough, and you might think their effects on your weight circumstance are negligible, but don't let appearances fool you. Sometimes the smallest bees give the biggest sting.

Leptin – The Master Hormone

Leptin is considered to be the master appetite-controlling hormone, as well as the most important factor in long-term weight management. Discovered in 1994, leptin was thought to be the key to weight-loss success, but much like any other miracle cure, it addressed only one small element in the factors contributing to weight gain, and it did not address other factors equally responsible for weight gain.

When we begin to lose weight, circulating levels of leptin, the starvation hormone, begin to drop and the body perceives the decrease in leptin as a loss of essential energy stored in the fat cells; as a result, it will instinctively act to protect the remaining fat stores. One way it does this is to slow the metabolism. You may feel the effects of a slowing metabolism as low energy and fatigue, but a slowing metabolism also means your body is not burning the calories you are consuming, which can bring your weight-loss efforts down to a crawl. Another way the body protects remaining fat stores is to limit the amount of energy used for non-vital functions. (I know I touched on this earlier, but it's worth repeating.)

The body's next response to decreasing levels of leptin is to bring those leptin levels back up to normal threshold levels – levels that are specific to your body – and restore what was lost as a result of your weight-loss efforts.

According to Dr. Robert H. Lustig, professor of pediatrics at the University of California, San Francisco, and a member of the Endocrine Society's Obesity Task Force, when your weight-loss efforts result in fat loss and the circulating levels of leptin decrease, the brain senses leptin levels have fallen below threshold and signals the stomach through the vagus nerve, thereby triggering your desire to feed. This has the goal of bringing the depleted levels of circulating leptin back up to normal threshold levels.[30] Once they are restored to normal threshold levels, the brain stops stimulating the vagus nerve and your desire to feed diminishes.

Thus, the key to minimizing the effects of decreasing leptin levels is not only to directly address the leptin itself but, also, to limit the effects of its enforcer – ghrelin.

Ghrelin – The Hunger Hormone

Ghrelin's nickname says it all: the hunger hormone. It is this little beasty that makes us hungry. Ghrelin is secreted by specialized cells in the fundus, or upper part of the stomach. It is also produced in small quantities by the brain, pancreas, and small intestine. Its job, plain and simple, is to get you to eat, to take on calories – to feed.

The hunger hormone is secreted when your stomach empties, increasing your desire to feed just before meals. But ghrelin doesn't just increase hunger or stimulate the relentless cravings experienced by dieters; it also promotes fat storage, which is trouble for dieters.

Whether you are dieting, fasting, over-restricting your caloric intake, or eating minute amounts of food in an attempt to lose weight, your ghrelin levels will rise and you will remain hungry. It is the body's attempt to replenish the circulating levels of leptin, and to restore any energy-storing fat reserves that might have been lost as a result of your weight-loss efforts. But ghrelin's efforts don't end with your diet; *Ghrelin levels increase after dieting.* And this explains much about why diet-induced weight loss can be difficult to maintain.[31] Minimizing the effects of leptin and ghrelin is essential to help sustain your weight loss and make your stabilization efforts work. Consuming healthy fats can help to minimize the effects of leptin, and consuming satiating foods throughout the day will limit the secretion of ghrelin. More on that a little further on.

The Good and Bad Bacteria

To say dietary standards have changed dramatically in the past fifty years would be an understatement. Busy schedules and increasingly hectic lifestyles lead us to consume increasing amounts of prepackaged, convenience, fast, and snack foods that weren't around a few decades ago. These contribute to the factors that influence our weight and waistlines.

For example, at least one in four people eat some form of fast food every day.[32] But our taste for these foods goes far beyond the convenience or flavor. Researchers believe that certain foods have an almost addictive quality. That is, when we consume them, our body releases "feel good" chemicals like dopamine, which researchers believe contributes to the addictive nature of certain foods. This could explain why we enjoy our comfort foods so much, how we grab them on the go or reach for them when we are feeling down or stressed. But it's not just the empty calories we get from eating these foods that presents the problem; it's also how they affect the body once we eat them.

There are over 100 trillion bacteria inside the stomach and intestine. There are both *positive* or good bacteria that support efficient digestion, a healthy immune system, and help to maintain the health, and function of the intestinal walls, and digestive system; and there are *negative* or bad gut bacteria that can cause a host of health and digestive issues if not kept in check. These issues include, but are not limited to, autoimmune disorders, infections, vitamin and mineral deficiencies, anemia, cravings, candidiasis, bowel disorders, food intolerances, osteoporosis, skin problems, and dairy allergies.

But that's not all the negative bacteria do. When negative bacteria proliferate, not only can they interfere with the body's ability to efficiently digest the foods we consume leading to weight gain, dietary bloat, and systemic inflammation, they can also negatively affect the intestinal wall over time, further influencing the efficiency with which we assimilate the vitamins, nutrients, and minerals the body needs to perform at optimal levels.

It might sound like throwing off the balance between good and bad bacteria would take some effort, but the truth is that the balance is delicate and can easily change from meal to meal, depending on the type of foods you consume. Something as simple as consuming a meal rich in simple carbohydrates like pasta can temporarily throw a punch to the gut biome, knocking it off balance. But it's not consuming carbs, or sugar-rich foods, once in a while we have to concern ourselves with. It is the repeated over-consumption of these foods that contributes to the weight-loss barriers, not to mention our expanding waistlines.

The average person consumes simple carbs three or more times each day, as well as two to three times the daily recommended amount of sugar.[33] Both supply a steady stream of nutrients that support an unhealthy gut biome – and all that goes with it.

Yet as harmful as consuming a lot of carbs and sugar-rich foods can be to the gut bacteria, its effects pale in comparison to other chemical and environmental factors to which we are exposed on a regular basis, including the widespread use of medications and antibiotics.

You may think that poor dietary habits are simply a matter of choice, but there might be more there than meets the eye when it comes to the foods we choose to consume. Evidence suggests that the negative gut bacteria have a secret weapon for influencing our dietary choices. That is, the negative gut bacteria thrive on starchy, sugar-rich foods, and to ensure they have a steady supply of the foods they like, they secrete chemical messengers that signal the brain to trigger cravings for these very foods. So, when we consume these foods, we are supporting the proliferation of negative gut bacteria, and the effects that come with them. The more you feed them what they want, the more you will crave those foods.

Remember this famous commercial, "Bet you just can't eat one"? Well, there's plenty of science to support why that is true when it comes to all sweet and starchy treats. When we eat them, we add fuel to the fire! But this doesn't mean you have to give up your favorite treats, and snacks forever. Rather, doing so might just be one of the reasons behind your weight-loss struggles.

The thought of never being able to enjoy a favorite food is one of the sustainability issues dieters have always faced. But despite the negative effects they have on our weight circumstance, and the fact that they support the proliferation of negative gut bacteria, these foods offer a certain amount of comfort and are actually part of an ongoing system of checks and balances in the digestive system. Understanding how these foods affect us, and knowing how to counter those effects is key to successful weight management.

IPS – Havoc in the Gut

Intestinal permeability syndrome, or IPS, is a condition that affects the intestinal walls, allowing the absorption of undigested food, bacteria, and toxins, which can wreak havoc on the body and immune system, and are responsible for causing a host of intestinal and other health disorders.

Research shows that IPS has been linked to the following:[34]

- Excessive sugar intake.
- Long-term use of Non-steroidal anti-inflammatory drugs (NSAIDs).
- Excessive alcohol intake.
- Deficiencies in vitamin A, vitamin D, and zinc.
- Chronic systemic inflammation (food-borne inflammation).
- Chronic stress.
- Poor gut health-disruption of the balance of good, and bad bacteria in the gut.
- Yeast overgrowth.

These formerly unknown adversaries of your weight management efforts disrupt the healthy balance of microorganisms in the stomach, and can lead to a decrease in the quantity and quality of gastric juices and digestive enzymes, resulting in inefficient digestion and assimilation of the foods we consume. In essence, they accelerate the degradation of the digestive system, and IPS can affect young, and old alike.

The key to minimizing their effects is to understand how they affect you, your weight loss, and your stabilization efforts. You get to know how to address these negatives with foods that equally support a healthy gut biome. Believe it or not, it's an easy fix.

Birthdays

The body's nutritional requirements remain relatively constant through-out life, but as we age, our ability to digest and absorb the foods we consume diminishes. Not only can the quantity and potency of the digestive enzymes and gastric juices like hydrochloric acid decrease reducing the efficiency of the digestive process, but the body's ability to absorb the vitamins, minerals, and macronutrients essential for optimal function also decreases.[35]

Imagine, if you will, the engine in your car. It converts the fuel you feed it into energy that makes your car run. When you first bought the car, you followed the recommendations provided in the owner's manual, and fueled the car with the best quality gasoline to get the best performance and gas mileage possible, and it ran flawlessly. You could feel the power of the engine when you drove down the street.

Now, jump forward ten years (twenty or thirty, in human years) and you find your car is running less than perfect. Parts are starting to wear out, and the effects of time and how you have used it are starting to show in its fuel efficiency and level of performance. It just doesn't have the get up and go it used to. So, you bring it to your mechanic, who recommends a can of octane booster – the car version of an energy drink – and it seems to help perk up the old engine a bit despite the occasional choke and sputter. But that effect lasts only so long, and you have to keep adding it to your gas tank.

Eventually, you realize your car requires something more than an energy boost, and you go back to your mechanic, who checks out your fuel system and finds everything looks pretty good until he looks at the fuel line, which he finds partially clogged and coated with debris. It's sediment from the *less expensive lower quality fuel* you have been using, which is restricting the amount of fuel energy your engine needs to run at its best.

Your mechanic asks if you have been using the right fuel, and you want to say yes, but know you have to be honest, so you tell him you've been feeding your car some low-grade gas because it was more convenient. Otherwise, you might have to put in extra time and effort to drive a few more blocks to get a better-quality gas for the car.

Your mechanic proceeds to clean out your gas line and adds a bottle of fuel system cleaner – the mechanic's version of a detox diet – to help clean out any gunk he can't see. You notice a substantial improvement in your car's performance, and you are thrilled, but both you and your mechanic know that eventually you're going to drift back to your old routine and start feeding your car the same discount brand low-grade gas that caused the problem to begin with just because it's a little more convenient.

This process is similar to what happens in the body. Your body requires fuel to function optimally, and this fuel comes from the foods you consume. The foods you consume are converted to the energy and nutrients essential for your body to function efficiently, and they are absorbed through the intestines – the body's fuel line – which over time can become damaged or coated with impurities that interfere with the supply of nutrients and energy.

This of course is an oversimplification of the process; however, it's a handy way to explain how over time the harmful bacteria, mucus, fecal material, fat globules, undigested and indigestible food particles, and toxins can impact the wall of the intestine and effect the efficiency with which you assimilate the nutrients your body requires.

Although the impurities and contaminants lining your car's fuel line will rarely lead to that fuel line's developing a leak, such is not the case with our intestine. Over time, exposure to contaminants, bacteria, chemicals, fertilizers, preservatives, irradiated foods, medications, and antibiotics can cause a subclinical condition called *intestinal permeability syndrome*, or IPS. It is also called "leaky gut" and is associated with gastrointestinal imbalance and assorted intestinal and systemic disorders.[36]

IPS affects our ability to absorb the vitamins, minerals, and nutrients our body requires to run efficiently, and it allows for the absorption of inefficiently digested food particles that can add weight, resulting in systemic inflammation. It also permits the absorption of harmful pathogens, bacteria, and parasites, and it enhances the uptake of toxic compounds into the blood stream, which can wreak havoc on the immune system, and can lead to autoimmune disorders, inflammatory joint disease, food allergies, and chronic skin conditions, just to name a few problems.

Unfortunately, time is not the only factor that affects the body's ability to efficiently process and assimilate the foods we consume. If it were, we might only see overweight adults, and not the increasing number of overweight and obese children, which are over 40 million strong. Today, one in three children and teens is overweight or obese.[37]

There are other factors that also negatively influence the body's ability to efficiently digest the foods we consume. Diet, lifestyle, the use of medications, drugs, alcohol, and the increasing amounts of environmental toxins and pollutants we are exposed to on a daily basis can have dramatic effects on the gastrointestinal system, which also affect your ability to maintain a healthier weight and waistline.

The Genetic Barriers

We've all heard someone play the genetics card. 'It's just the way I am." "Everyone in my family is like this." And that may be true. You may come from a family in which the majority of people are overweight. But that doesn't necessarily mean your weight circumstance is all the result of genetics, or that you can't improve upon the perfection that is you.

When we talk about genetics in regard to weight loss, we are not speaking about those combinations of genes that are passed down through ancestral lines and that provide us with the physical characteristics that yield our unique look, like facial features, height or physical stature, hair, eye and skin color, skeletal structure, or the size of your digits, feet, ears, nose, and lips. What we are talking about are the fat genes: FTO, IRX3, and IRX 5, and their variants.

FTO (alpha-ketoglutarate-dependent dioxygenase) is also known as the "fat gene." This is a relatively new discovery. It is a protein associated with overweight and obesity that was discovered in 2006. Studies have shown that certain variants of FTO can result in higher levels of ghrelin – the hunger hormone – and higher levels of IRX3, and IRX5. As you may remember, ghrelin triggers hunger and supports long-term fat storage.

The IRX3, and IRX5 genes have been shown to support the conversion of fat from the foods we ingest into unhealthy "visceral or white fat" that stores lipids, or the unsightly fat that accumulates around the stomach, neck, hips, and thighs, instead of healthy "brown fat" that provides the body with a ready source of energy to burn.[38]

Sadly, most dieters who play the genetics card do so because they have failed to see the results they desire from their weight-loss efforts, and may be ready to throw in the towel on weight-loss altogether. But lack of success alone, or temporary success, does not mean you are predisposed to be overweight or obese.

Surprisingly, it's relatively simple to address the effects these genes have on your overall weight circumstance. You see, the fat genes FTO, IRX3, and IRX5 have an on/off switch of sorts. It's a fat switch that you can control simply by increasing the amounts of polyphenol-rich foods in your diet and limiting your intake of starchy carbs and sugar-rich foods until you have optimized your body's ability to process and assimilate those foods.

The foods that can turn off your fat switch are not exotic, new weight-loss miracle diet foods; they are foods people eat every day, and you can buy at any market. They the brightly colored fruits and vegetables that contain high concentrations of antioxidant-rich phytonutrients. Here are just a few.

• Blackberries	• Red grapes
• Red raspberries	• Artichoke hearts
• Blueberries	• Flaxseed meal
• Strawberries	• Dark chocolate
• Sweet cherries	• Chestnuts
• Plums	• Black tea
• Pure apple Juice	• Green tea
• Apples	• Coffee
• Pure pomegranate Juice	• Whole-grain rye bread
• Black olives	• Hazelnuts
• Spinach	• Red wine
• Pecans	• Cocoa powder
• Black beans	• Red onions
• Leafy green veggies	• Broccoli

Polyphenol-rich foods can turn your fat-storing switch off and turn your fat-burning switch on when they are added to your diet. They not only prevent the conversion of the foods you eat into unhealthy white fat but also help convert that unhealthy white fat into the healthy brown fat your body uses for energy. Adding these foods to your diet is a win-win for you.

The Psychological Barriers

Have you ever wondered why you feel and think the things you do before, during, and after a diet? Did you ever think this may not be by happenstance, that there's a reason why we think and feel the way we do?

The psychological factors contributing to this barrier have nothing to do with psychopathology, or any abnormal thought processes that result in disorders of the mind, like anxiety, depression, bipolar disorders, substance abuse, or the eating disorders some people develop. These are serious problems far beyond the scope and content of this text. But the psychological barriers dieters can address here are the paradigms, beliefs, and behaviors that influence our thought processes, decisions, and actions as they relate to our weight loss and overall eating behaviors. These are the deeply rooted behaviors we've learned and practiced since early childhood.

The brain is one of the most powerful computers on the face of the earth. It processes upwards of 400 billion bits of information per second,[39] and outside of monitoring and controlling every aspect and function of your body, its purpose is to *protect and preserve* your life against any and all perceived threats, whether real or imagined. To do this, it relies on instinctual behaviors and reflexes passed down ancestral lines, as well as the knowledge you have gathered from years of education, personal experience, observations, rituals, routine, and traditions practiced during your lifetime.

Imagine you were born and raised in a tropical climate. Early one spring, you made your first trip north to visit friends in Maine, and you and your friends decided to take a walk through a local park. During the walk one of your friends sees the pond is still frozen from the cold winter months, and knowing it would be something new and fun for you, invites you to run and slide across the ice.

Your friend shows you how it's done, but you're a little nervous, wondering if it's something you should try. Having lived your entire life in a tropical climate, you've never seen an ice covered pond before, much less walked or slid on it. But it looks like fun, so you gather your courage, run to the edge of the pond, and begin to slide your way out to the middle of the pond where your friend is standing. And just before you get there, you hear a thunderous cracking sound underfoot echoing across the pond. Your heart begins to pound, and both you and your wide-eyed friend run off the ice.

This is instinctual behavior, a response to an unsettling loud noise that engages our fight-or-flight reflex. Somewhere along our ancestral lines, we've learned to associate certain loud sounds with danger. You'd never heard the sound before, but instinctively you knew it was something to be alarmed about.

Now let's say, you're on the same walk, but this time you have been on an ice-covered pond before, and like me, you've actually fallen through the ice. When your friend invites you to slide out on the ice, the little voice inside your head reminds you of the dangers of doing so. You might in an instant mentally relive the experience of falling through the ice. You remember the panic you felt when the ice cracked and you fell through. The smell of muddy pond water, and the bone-chilling cold you felt when you hit the water. You can feel the weight of layers of water-soaked clothing pulling you down as you try to claw your way up and over the cracking ice, out of the frigid waters. This is the mind's attempt to protect you from doing something potentially dangerous, by using a learned experience to influence your current decision on whether or not to slide out onto the ice.

The mind works in a similar way when it comes to your weight-loss efforts, but in the case of weight loss, it's not the flight-or-fight reflex. It's a protective mechanism developed over the course of countless generations, and its job is to protect you against the possibility of starvation.

The mind perceives weight loss as the loss of vital energy stored in fat, which in the past and to our body's programming, is a bad thing. To our distant ancestors, fat was not the inconvenience it is today. It was essential for survival, and building the body's fat stores during times when food is relatively abundant was necessary, so we have it when it isn't otherwise available.

Fat insulates and protects our vital organs, provides warmth and energy during lean times, and plays a crucial role in protecting us from the possibility of starvation. Gaining weight was once so essential to survival that it became a part of the body's operating system. Alas, it functions today much as it did for our ancestors, which is why you may notice you tend to gain weight in the fall and winter months.

It might seem strange to you, thinking that your mind could actually believe you are starving when actually you are fortunate to live with such abundance. But it does. The mind responds to the information it is programmed with, which is the knowledge and instinctual behavior we have inherited from our ancestors.

The abundance we take for granted today did not exist a hundred years ago and earlier. Our more distant ancestors consumed only what they could kill, catch, scavenge, or gather. Just like any other animal, they were dependent on seasonal foods, and their hunting, fishing, and gathering skills. An abundant supply of food just wasn't guaranteed. As a result, our body has been programmed to perceive weight loss as potentially life-threatening. It will work against your conscious desire and your efforts to lose weight, and this is part of why you feel, think, and do what you do before, during, and after dieting.

It's not uncommon for seasoned dieters to experience a certain amount of trepidation before beginning another round of dieting. Once the thought of beginning another diet pops into our heads, we are reminded of what the next few weeks or months will bring: the restrictions, compromises, constant hunger, cravings, expense, stress, agitation, and moodiness. Adding to that is the frustration that follows when those hard-earned results begin to reverse themselves. Reminding you of the difficulties of dieting is the mind's way of using prior experience to prevent you from stepping out on the ice.

Have you ever wondered why, when you are dieting you are always hungry, craving certain foods, even after a meal? Or why the hunger and cravings get stronger the longer you continue to diet? Or why your senses suddenly tune into everything and anything related to food? You may have walked passed the same burger place, bakery, or restaurant a thousand times, without a second thought. But as soon as you begin to diet, you are suddenly aware of the sound and smell of something sizzling on a grill, or the aroma of fresh-baked bread, pastries, cakes, and pies filling the air.

And why, when your diet finally comes to an end, do you continue to crave foods you know will pack on the pounds? Why is it you rationalize allowing yourself to indulge in them more frequently than you know you should, especially when you consider the weeks or months of effort you just put into shedding those unwanted pounds and inches? We've all thought it: "One bite can't hurt." Besides, we can always go back on the diet for a few more days…

\This is the body and mind working to put an end to your weight-loss efforts. Understanding why you do, think, and feel these things goes a long way toward helping you achieve lasting results.

Wit and Willpower – Let the Games Begin

I don't profess to be an expert in psychology; in fact, I am far from it. My interests lay only in understanding why we do, feel, and think the things we do when dieting, and in understanding how the body and mind respond to weight loss. The best way to understand how paradigms, beliefs, and behaviors influence our weight-loss and stabilization efforts is to understand how the mind can work either for or against those efforts.

Sigmund Freud used an iceberg to explain the levels of mind, and how each level works to influence our thoughts, decisions, and actions.[40] According to Freud, there are three levels of the mind: conscious, subconscious, and unconscious.

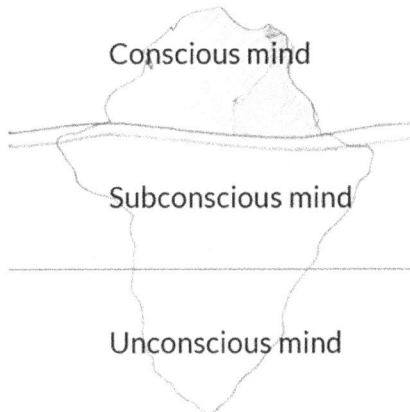

Conscious mind

Subconscious mind

Unconscious mind

The Conscious Mind

The conscious mind is the tip of the iceberg, and it contains what we are aware of now. For example, you are aware you are reading this book.

If you feel hungry, you become aware of it and can get something to eat – or you may decide to hold off. This is the frontline for dieters or anyone else wishing to question and/or change a behavior. It's only here that you can decide what, when, and if you should eat something to satisfy your cravings – or to hold off in continuance of your weight-loss efforts.

The conscious mind is the one place we can modify our eating behaviors and address the thoughts, feelings, and emotions associated with dieting. It is the only part of the mind we have access to, and it is only while we are awake. Alas, that puts our weight-loss efforts at a disadvantage. It is here that we battle the constant hunger and cravings. It is here that we put off the temptation to stray from our weight-loss efforts. And it is here that we can confront the paradigms, beliefs, and behaviors we have regarding the foods we eat, how we eat them, and how we should lose weight, especially if that's not the way we've been taught all along.

Dieting, taken at face value, seems simple enough: just cut calories, and we'll lose weight – right? Oh, if it were only that simple. We've all seen how well that works in providing lasting results.

When we consciously decide to go on a diet, it's not just a battle of will-power. We are not simply competing against our ability to sustain restricted caloric intake long enough to reach our weight-loss goals. We are entering into a contest of wit and wills against an opponent equally intelligent and more cunning than we realize. It's an opponent programmed to enforce instinctual behaviors and preserve life, as well as protect us from danger, whether that danger is real or perceived – the subconscious mind.

The Subconscious Mind

The second level of the mind is the subconscious. It comprises the bulk of the iceberg and sits just beneath the water's surface, out of sight and out of mind. It is a reservoir of learned behaviors and stored information gathered from your formal education, personal experience, training, family rituals, daily routines, traditions, and observations of your environment, which you are not presently aware of.

As you are reading this you're probably not thinking of where you left your keys, but now that I mentioned them, you know where they are or where you should look for them. The mere mention of your keys results in something you were unaware in the prior moment being now brought to conscious awareness.

The subconscious is the little voice in your head that says, "Oh, yeah… that's where my keys are." It's the voice of reason, which tells us if something is safe or dangerous, right or wrong, and whether or not we should act on conscious thoughts or decisions – like sliding out on an ice-covered pond, tasting some strange new exotic food, or going on a diet.

It uses the information gathered over your lifetime to influence your thoughts, decisions, and actions. And in the case of weight loss and dieting, once you make the conscious decision to lose weight, your subconscious will be there to remind you of just how much you dislike dieting.

We are creatures of habit. We've eaten the same foods for breakfast, lunch, and dinner our entire lives; and to our mind, eating three times per day is normal, as are the types and combinations of foods we consume. Now, you decide to go on a diet. You radically change your diet, reduce your caloric intake, eliminate the majority of foods you've consumed your entire life, and expect your body to accept the change without a fight. *Not Happening!*

The body doesn't like change, and it will use every resource available to bring you back to what you have trained it to believe is normal for you. And the subconscious mind is leading the charge.

In Chapter 2, you may recall the discussion about how it was getting harder and harder to lose weight, with each successive diet making the dieter seek more aggressive approaches to weight loss. This happens because the subconscious mind has learned what poker players would call a "tell." This is a change in behavior, giving other players clues as to your assessment of your hand. In this case, the other player is your subconscious mind.

In weight loss, the tell is restricting caloric intake over a longer period of time than what is normal for you. When you begin to restrict your caloric intake, chemical messengers signal the brain that your caloric intake has decreased, which triggers the mind to stimulate hunger and cravings. It's the body's attempt to get you to consume more calories. The longer you restrict your caloric intake, the harder the body will work against your weight-loss efforts. Why?

Because we are programmed to store fat, and not to release it.

The mind is a most cunning adversary. But it's not infallible – it can be defeated if you know what to eat and how to eat it, so as to minimize the effects of the chemical messengers signaling the brain.

The Unconscious Mind

The third level of mind is the unconscious. It is represented by the base of the iceberg, deep underwater. The unconscious mind holds information that is inaccessible to us. Our deepest fears, emotions, instincts, and base desires reside in the unconscious; and it is believed by some, to be the primary source of our behavior.[41]

The unconscious is home to the body's survival programming: the fight-or-flight reflex, infant suckling reflex, the mating reflex, and most especially here, the starvation response, or reflex that works to prevent the loss of fat and protect us from the possibility of starvation.

Our ancestors, much like nonmigratory animals, were driven to build fat stores to help them survive the long winter months, and it is this survival mechanism that continues to influence our weight circumstance today.

You see it every fall, when just like clockwork the weight scales across the country begin to climb. As the seasons change, so do the foods we consume. Lighter, cooler summer fare is replaced by increased amounts of calorie-dense body-warming comfort foods. But what seems to be nothing more than simple convention to us is in reality an instinctual behavior to build fat reserves and energy stores for the winter season.

Although we cannot readily access or change such instinctual behaviors, we can consciously work to modify our eating behaviors, without having to give up the foods we enjoy. In doing so, not only can we accelerate the weight-loss process but we can also stabilize our post-diet weight by minimizing the workings of the mind and relax the chemical messengers responsible for triggering the starvation reflex when dieting.

Addressing learned behaviors, paradigms, and beliefs begins with questioning them if they have a place in your life today, and assessing whether they are helping or hindering your weight-management efforts. For example, you might question which would benefit you most: waiting for the elevator or taking the stairs? Here are some other questions you can ask:

- Is eating three times a day the best way to provide my body with the nutrients, and energy it needs?
- How do the foods I'm eating affect my weight?
- How do artificial sweeteners affect me?

- Is there a better way to get the most nutritional benefit from my meals?

- Am I eating the right combinations of foods?

- Is cutting calories the best way for me to lose weight?

- What medications do I take on a regular basis? How do they affect my body, and what can I do to minimize unwanted side effects?

- How often do I eat takeout – fast, processed, and or junk foods?

- What snacks do I eat before bedtime, and what effect do they have on weight loss?

Now, these may not be the exact questions you might come up with, but they are questions you'll want the answers to because each answer influences your ability to maintain and stabilize a healthier weight and waistline.

When you begin to question your daily routines, practices, and habits, especially those regarding your eating behaviors, you might be surprised to see just how many of the things you are doing can be improved upon – and some may no longer be applicable to your lifestyle today.

In order to modify these behaviors, you need to replace or update them much as you would update the software on your computer, tablet, or smartphone. But replacing outdated information and practices with current information and practices is sometimes easier said than done.

Studies show that new habits can be formed in as little as a few days. Others suggest that the length of time it takes to change a habit is 66 days; however, the more complex or deeply embedded the habit, belief, or behavior is, the longer it takes to change it.[42] Some changes, like dieting, can take upwards of nine months, which is far beyond the average dieter's ability to sustain weight-loss efforts.

You see, as mentioned several times already, your conscious decision to lose weight goes against the body's programming to maintain normalcy. You know you're only trying to lose a few pounds, but your mind doesn't know that, and there is no way for you to convince it otherwise. Regardless of how you came to be overweight, your body, and mind sees this status as normal. This doesn't mean it's considered normal or healthy by medical standards, of course. It simply means the body has adapted to that excess weight in one way or another.

The body does not know the textbook definition of a healthy weight. It has no idea where you should be on a BMI chart. The mind only responds to the signals it receives from the body, and as far as it is concerned, a decrease in leptin, whether that decrease is in someone who is 5 pounds overweight or 55 pounds overweight, will trigger the same protective response.

The problem we face is, when we pit our conscious desire to lose weight against the workings of the mind and body, it's much like playing a game of chess against a grand master. To further the metaphors, your subconscious has the home field advantage because it can work against your weight-loss efforts 24/7/365, whereas you can only work on weight loss during the hours you're awake.

Now, we may not be able to change our instincts or the survival mechanisms that have protected us for millennia, but in understanding how the game is played, we can modify our behavior to work in favor of our weight-loss efforts, without the radical lifestyle changes or dietary restrictions we've previously used to inefficiently manage our weight and waistlines.

The Environmental Barriers

There are a number of major contributors to the environmental barrier that influence our ability to maintain a healthier weight, including, but not limited to, the eating behaviors we learn as children in the family environment; the effects stress has on the body; one's level of activity at work, home, and play; the influence the media and advertising on our eating behaviors; and the effects antibiotics, environmental toxins, and pollutants have on the body.

"You are a product of your environment." This quote, attributed to the late W. Clement Stone, was used in his work to help those seeking to improve their lives. His message was that each person should survey his or her environment to determine whether the environment is conducive to achieving personal goals, dreams, designs, and desires; if it is not, he or she should act to find an environment that will best help develop the mindset to achieve those goals and objectives. Stone wisely advised his followers to analyze life in terms of their environment.[43] His advice holds true for managing your weight, as well.

But what constitutes the environment? The environmental barrier is a playing field in a constant state of change. Stress levels are on the rise and physical activity is declining. The three-square-meal per day standard most adults were raised with is moving toward three squares plus a late-night snack. Add in the effects that chemicals, medications, and antibiotics have on the body, not to mention the increasing number chemical additives, artificial sweeteners, preservatives, coloring, and stabilizers used in our foods; the fertilizers, pesticides, sewerage sludge, irradiation, and chemicals used to grow, protect or ripen the fruits, and vegetables we consume; the chemicals, drugs, hormones, and antibiotics used on livestock we consume, and the eggs, dairy, and other food products that come from them; and the Billions of tons of chemical toxins released into the environment every year.[44] These present a most formidable adversary to weight-loss efforts.

The degree to which each factor contributes to the environmental barrier will differ depending on your geographical location, family life, employment, and lifestyle. Fortunately, much of the influence these factors have on our bodies can be offset or minimized simply by adjusting your dietary intake.

The Family Dynamic

As children, we learn and develop many of the habits that later govern our eating behaviors as adults. These are behaviors that become increasingly difficult to change as we grow older. If we are raised in a family environment that supports healthy eating habits and activity levels, it is likely that we will continue those habits through adulthood. Conversely, if we are raised in a family environment where activity is limited and the motto at mealtime is *abbondanza*, and/or eating fast-foods, take-out, and junk foods is the rule, we will likely carry this behavior into adulthood along with our plus-sized pants.

Unfortunately, the family dynamic is trending toward consuming less healthy whole foods and more take-out, prepacked, and fast-foods. Singles and families alike are seeking easy mealtime options to ease the stress of hectic lifestyles. That trend is taking its toll on our weight and waistlines. These foods are generally higher in unhealthy fats, carbs, and sugars, and often contain chemical stabilizers and preservatives that can kill bacteria (good and bad), as well as negatively influence the digestive tract.

The statistics speak for themselves. Global overweight, and obesity levels for adults and children, have doubled and tripled in as many decades. Many countries are pointing their fingers at the $300+ billion-dollar convenience food industry, and the $100+ billion-dollar junk-food industry, accusing them of getting fat on our dollars while we get fat on their food. Countries traditionally known for their healthy, active lifestyles are reporting staggering increases in childhood obesity, some with upwards of 44% of children reported as overweight or obese.[45]

Earlier we covered the best way to evaluate the behaviors and paradigms influencing our thoughts, decisions, and actions. Well, when it comes to improving your weight circumstance, your eating behaviors and habits are a good place to start. For example, one of the most common eating practices the world over is that of three square meals per day. Interestingly enough, this practice was not developed because it was healthier to eat this way but, rather, was born of greed and envy.[46] The practice continues today more as a matter of social convention and convenience, despite numerous articles and studies suggesting that eating three square meals per day is neither the best nor the healthiest way to provide the body with the nutrients and energy required.[47] Continuing to follow this paradigm is actually contributing to the overweight and obesity epidemic.

Eating three square meals per day is a social convention that goes against our natural instinct to eat when hungry. Newborns get hungry on average every one and a half to three hours. By one or two months old, they're feeding seven to nine times per day.[48] As they get older, parents wean them off the bottle, onto baby foods, then onto whole foods, which is where we stop following our natural instincts to feed when hungry.

It's not likely you will eliminate this practice from your life; however, you can easily modify this behavior to improve the effectiveness of your weight-loss efforts by eating more frequently throughout the day.

Don't Stress About It

Stress is the brain's and body's response to any demand, whether physical, emotional or otherwise, and with today's hectic lifestyles, there's plenty of it to go around. Stress can be found in most every aspect of life. We have stress at work, home, school, and with friends and family members. There are emotional, physical, marital, financial, and social stresses that affect us physically, as well as emotionally.

In small quantities stress, isn't all bad. It can help motivate us to accomplish a task or move us to correct undesirable situations. But the cumulative effects of daily stress can take its toll on the body.[49] Stress affects every system in the body, causing physical, emotional, cognitive, and behavioral symptoms. Living with stress not only adds to your waistline but can also interfere with your ability to lose and maintain a healthy weight.[50]

Unfortunately, stress has become so commonplace that it often goes unnoticed. It is perceived as a normal part of everyday life. It is another of those things we can't see that not only works against our weight-loss efforts but also can dramatically impact our overall health and wellbeing. Every two seconds, seven people die as a direct result of stress, and upwards of 75% of doctor office visits are for stress-related ailments.[51] The question is: How does stress influence your weight circumstance?

Stress causes the body to secrete a number of chemicals associated with our fight-or-flight reflex: epinephrine, norepinephrine, and cortisol. In the short term, these chemicals work to provide us with the extra energy needed to perform an energy-expending task or to respond to potentially dangerous or harmful situations. They are responsible for the rapid heartbeat and surge of energy you feel when startled by someone or something, but when elevated for extended periods of time, they can cause a number of serious health issues,[52] and result in overweight and obesity.

Of the three, cortisol is the one dieters need concern themselves with most because cortisol is the chemical equivalent of public enemy number one for your weight and waistline. Cortisol is known to increase the appetite and cravings for high-calorie foods. It promotes high blood sugar levels and the suppression of insulin, which can turn the occasional indulgence or overeating into a bad habit. It aids in the growth of fat cells and promotes visceral (white) fat storage, and has been shown to have a direct relationship to increased caloric intake, as well as contributing to a host of digestive disorders.[53]

To manage the effects of cortisol, you can start by finding ways to manage your stress. Exercise is one form of stress release (but don't overdo it). The body perceives intense workouts also as stress, which increases circulating levels of cortisol. Light exercise will help alleviate stress, and will result in the production of endorphins – the bodies painkiller. It also helps you get a good night's sleep.

You can also trigger the secretions of stress-relieving endorphins with meditation, acupuncture, or by getting a massage. Simple deep-breathing exercises similarly help the body produce endorphins. Have you ever sighed deeply after watching a suspense-filled movie scene? It's the same thing. That's a calming effect used to offset the stress you just experienced watching the movie.

In recent years the use of essential oils has rapidly increased following reports that they can be incredibly effective at minimizing the effects of daily stress. The aromatic molecules can pass straight through the blood-brain barrier affecting changes in mood and minimizing tension, and lowering overall stress levels.[54] Lavender, cinnamon, cedar, jasmine, lime, grapefruit, and eucalyptus essential oils are just a few of those helping countless numbers of people to ease the tensions of the day.

Essential oils can be effective when used around the home, and office; however, they are most effective when used during your down time, or the time of day when you can escape the rigors of life and enjoy some peace and quiet.[55]

Physical Activity

Mention physical activity to anyone on a diet, and the first thing they will likely think of is exercise. But as important as exercise is to maintaining an active, healthy lifestyle, it is not essential to your weight-loss efforts.

That may come as a surprise to you, but during the two-month period when I dropped 40 pounds, I did so while sedentary, with zero exercise. My activities were limited to going from bed, to a chair, and back again two, three, and sometimes four times per day. I was able to do so because I learned how to easily address the barriers, blocks, and changes that were interfering with my ability to lose weight, and in doing so, I was able to optimize my ability to process and assimilate the food I was eating into fat-burning energy.

Now, I'm not saying you shouldn't exercise. What I am saying is, if for whatever reason you are presently unable to exercise, you can improve, even accelerate, the results achieved through your weight-loss efforts simply by optimizing your body's ability to process and assimilate the foods you consume.

Does this mean you will lose 40 pounds as quickly as I did? Not necessarily. Depending on your particular circumstance; your starting weight; the number and degree of barriers, blocks, and changes you need to address; and your diligence in doing so, you could lose the same, less, or even more weight than I was able to. The latter is because you have the ability to do something I couldn't at the time – you can move about freely throughout the day, which expends energy, and you have the option to increase your energy expenditure and calorie burn by exercising. An option I didn't have.

There are four levels of physical activity used to describe individual lifestyles.[56] The vast majority of people will pass through three of the four levels as we transition from childhood to active adult life.

As children, we're usually very active and readily burn the calories we consume. As we pass through our pre-teens and teens, we remain relatively active until we reach our late teens, when our focus turns to college matriculation and/or joining the working world. In our early and mid-twenties, our focus shifts to pursuing our careers and to developing relationships, which may eventually lead to starting our own families. By this time, physical activity levels may have dropped upwards of 75 % from where they were when we were kids.

As adults we are either *sedentary*, whereby we are not physically active at work or home, and get no formal exercise; or we are *lightly active*, whereby our daily routine involves non-exertional physical activity at work and home, and no formal exercise; or we are *moderately* active, whereby we are active throughout the day. At this level, we might have an average interest in health and fitness, and get some type of formal exercise three to five times per week.

The final level is the *very active*, whereby we go nonstop at work, home, and play. Our interest in health and fitness may be above average, we follow a structured exercise routine, often daily. We take the stairs over the elevator, walk instead of ride, and are usually somewhat nutritionally conscious, despite the fact that our frenetic nature tends us to burning calories as quickly as we consume them.

As you take a survey of the barriers, blocks, and changes restraining your weight-loss efforts, you will want to assess your current activity level so you can modify and streamline your weight-loss efforts to improve and/or accelerate your results.

The Prescription Is...

Antibiotics and other orally ingested medications are at the top of the list of environmental influencers affecting weight and waistlines. The widespread use of antibiotics and other medications are a common part of everyday life, with over 42 billion daily doses of antibiotics taken annually. It is estimated that by 2030, that number will increase 200% to 128 billion daily doses annually.[57] Alarming!

There's no question that antibiotics and other medications play an important role in helping to keep us healthy, and for some, keeping them alive. Penicillin alone is credited with saving the lives of over 200 million people since it was discovered by Sir Alexander Fleming in 1928.[58] Penicillin, its derivatives and other antibiotics will continue to have their place in the world for generations to come; however, as with everything else in life, there is a cause and effect when using antibiotics.

As important as antibiotics are in keeping us healthy, they wreak havoc on the digestive system and the body's ability to efficiently process and assimilate the foods we consume into the macronutrients and energy required by the body to function at optimal levels.[59] Taking antibiotics when we are sick or have an infection comes as naturally to us as taking aspirin, Advil, or Tylenol when we have a headache; however, doing so can disrupt the balance of good and bad bacteria in your gastrointestinal tract for months at a time.

Numerous studies have been conducted on the effects of antibiotic administration, and dysbiosis, or the change in composition and function of the gastrointestinal system that results from taking antibiotics, and each suggests a marked change in the healthy balance of the bacterial flora contained within the stomach.[60] Antibiotics work to either kill or prevent bacteria from multiplying. Unfortunately, unlike our computers, smartphones, and televisions, antibiotics are not smart. They can't single out one type of pathogen, recognize it as the problem, and eliminate it. This means they can't differentiate between the good bacteria in your stomach and digestive tract that help you to efficiently digest the foods you consume and the bad bacteria that negatively impact your health and digestive abilities.

When antibiotics are used, not only do they disrupt the healthy balance of positive and negative bacteria in the digestive track, they also allow for opportunistic organisms in the stomach and intestine to flourish in the absence of healthy levels of positive gut bacteria that normally would hold them in check.[61] Negative gut bacteria produce chemicals like propionic acid, which contribute to triggering cravings, hunger, and systemic inflammation that affects the body's ability to burn calories, among other things.[62] What this means for dieters, or anyone else struggling with weight issues is, weight gain.

As much as antibiotics influence the weight circumstance of adults, their effect on children can be much more profound. Numerous studies conducted around the world have shown the use of antibiotics in early childhood correlates with excessive weight gain in later childhood.[63]

Now, there's no doubt there is a small percentage of people struggling with weight issues who have never had the need to take antibiotics in their lives – and if you are one of them, Congratulations! – but that doesn't mean you are exempt from the adverse effects of antibiotics and other medications. Because even though you may have never used antibiotics, it's likely you are exposed to them on a daily basis through the foods you handle and consume, and through the people you come in contact with.

You see, whereas we take antibiotics after we become ill, the ranchers raising the livestock that are used as a food source administer antibiotics to prevent illness and the spread of diseases common to livestock. And they don't only use antibiotics to protect livestock from harmful bacteria and pathogens, they also use low doses of antibiotics to fatten up livestock.[64] Ranchers have long known what dieters don't know. When they administer low doses of antibiotics to livestock, they fatten up without having to give them more food.[65] Hmmm? Sounds familiar.

The problem with this situation is that we are then exposed to low levels of antibiotics by consuming the products produced by these animals: the eggs, milk, cheese, and other dairy products, as well as the meat and poultry. Learning to properly address the adverse effects of medications we take for illness, and that we also ingest when consuming nonorganic animal food products, is essential to maintaining a healthy balance of bacteria in the gut.

Today it's not uncommon for doctors and pharmacists to recommend eating yogurt, drinking kefir or using some form of probiotic support, to help restore healthy levels of positive bacteria in the gut that have been decimated as a result of antibiotics, but simply taking probiotics or ingesting yogurt while you are taking medications is not enough. The imbalance of positive and negative bacteria that results from taking antibiotics and other medications can last for weeks – even months – making it increasingly difficult for you to achieve your weight-loss goals, especially during fall and winter months when cold and flu season promotes increased use of such medications.

Chemicals, Toxins, and Pollutants

Another contributor to the environmental barrier influencing your weight and waistline are the chemicals, toxins, and pollutants we are exposed to on a daily basis.

Environmental toxins (ETs) are those chemicals, toxins, and pollutants we are exposed to every day – Know it or not. We'll be getting more into them when we cover the environmental barriers; however, it is important to understand that environmental toxins contribute to and accelerate the effects of those physical barriers – and our ability to process and assimilate the foods we consume into fat-burning energy.

You may be under the impression that you are not exposed to environmental toxins because you don't work in or live near an industry that deals with chemicals, manufacturing, or energy production. But the truth is, it doesn't matter anymore where you live or work – you are exposed to toxins every day, and have been since the day you were born.

Your exposure comes from both internal and external sources. External sources of toxins can be found in the products you use on a daily basis in your home. They are found in the antibiotics and medications we use. In the beauty products used on your face and body. In the fabrics used for carpeting, bedding, and clothing, and in the materials used to make mattresses, furniture, and household appliances. Environmental toxins are found in the water we drink, the air we breathe, and the soil we grow our foods in. But don't panic. The body can deal with most toxins with a little help. It's the environment I'd be more concerned with.

Just about everything we consume, unless it is certified 100% organic or antibiotic free, has been exposed to some form of chemical toxin or pollutant, whether intentional or not. Filling the shelves of over thirty-six thousand grocery stores, thirty thousand plus food processing plants, over fifty thousand fast food chains, countless mom, and pop stores, and over six hundred-sixteen thousand restaurants is an immense undertaking.[66] In order to ensure a healthy supply of fruits and vegetables make it to the shelves of these stores, the processing plants, and restaurants, it is necessary to take measures to protect those food sources, and also protect us from harmful bacteria, insects, parasites, and other harmful pathogens that negatively impact our food supplies.

Farmers are under constant pressure to keep up with the demand for fresh foods, and in order to do so they must use chemicals, fertilizers, and pesticides to grow and protect their crops. Produce imported from other parts of the world are harvested before fully matured, and sprayed with chemical compounds to help them ripen during transport. Then they are sprayed with pesticides to kill any and all insects, pathogens, and bacteria that could potentially harm us, and are often irradiated as a final measure to protect us and to prevent the introduction of new pathogens and parasites that could decimate local and national crops.

As necessary as these measures are, the chemicals, fertilizers, and pesticides used by farmers to protect us and our foods, and the preservatives, coloring, stabilizers, and flavor enhancers used by food companies producing the tons of processed pre-packaged foods we consume daily, all contribute to influencing your weight circumstance.

The internal toxins we are exposed to come in the form of by-products of digestion, which are given off by certain foods we ingest. And it's not just the foods you might expect. It's not only the carbs and snack foods; it's also the frozen foods, canned and processed foods, genetically modified foods, and foods that are mass produced, flavored, dyed, and preserved.[67]

Finding it hard to believe? Recently the Environmental Working Group tasked Eurofins, a nationally recognized lab with testing food products containing oats, including children's cereals, breakfast bars, and granola. They found potentially toxic levels of a chemical called glyphosate, a carcinogen linked to non-Hodgkin's lymphoma in all but two of forty-five popular oat products.

Glyphosate is a systemic herbicide, which means it is taken up into every part of the plant, including the parts fed to livestock and those we consume, and according to the U.S. Geological Survey, over 250 million pounds of it is sprayed on crops each year.[68]

Understanding that certain foods and environmental toxins contribute to the physical barriers influencing your weight-loss efforts is the first step toward being able to address them. And this can be accomplished simply by adjusting your dietary intake to include whole foods and products that support healthy digestive function and weight stabilization.

Sensory-Media Cues

When you consider all the things that influence your weight, the last thing you would probably think of are the endless streams of advertisements you see, hear, and read. We see them so often that we pay them little, to no attention. But do you know how advertising works to affect or otherwise influence your thoughts, decisions, and actions?

There is an art, and a science, to advertising, and those who do it well are compensated equally well by the companies that hire them. The sole purpose of advertising and marketing is to get you, the consumer, to buy whatever product is being offered, now or in the future. And to do that, savvy marketers, some of whom could sell sand to someone in the desert, use every trick in the book.

They use trends, psychology, and statistical data gathered every time a consumer makes a purchase in their marketing strategies. They conduct marketing surveys to determine what people think and feel about products being offered, and do a thorough market analysis. They learn what, when, where, and how to present the product to you before developing an orchestrated plan of attack designed to get you to buy it – but I'm sure that comes as no surprise.

However, have you ever wondered why there are so many late-night food and chain restaurant commercials aired just before bedtime? Marketers know your mind is most open to suggestion just before you fall asleep, and this is the perfect time to get their message into your head. What's that little trick parents use to ease the minds of children before bedtime? Repeatedly tell them not to dream about puppies and bunnies, and they can't help but do so. It's the same principle. In fact, the late Earl Nightingale of Nightingale-Conant developed a "Learn While You Sleep Program" decades ago using this principle. It was one I used to help me ace an organic chemistry final (not one of my strongest subjects).

Marketers know the mind is most receptive to receiving information just before we wake up and just before we fall into deep sleep. If one of the last things you see on television before you fall asleep is someone pushing toward you on the screen a plate of sizzling fajitas, a bacon cheeseburger, or a plate of nachos piled high, covered with meat and melted cheese, you might wake up craving one of them and plan a trip to a favorite chain restaurant that day, or in the near future. You might also notice an increase in these commercials just before mealtime, when you are hungry and more open to suggestion.

There are a number of effective methods used to influence our dietary habits, but not all advertisements are geared toward things as enjoyable as food. Many products and services promoted are things we don't like, or even dread the thought of having to use or do, like weight-loss and dieting products. For instance, I don't think there's a person on the planet looking forward to the next time he or she has to go on a diet. So, how do advertisers sell you on committing your precious time, effort, and hard-earned money on products and programs to lose the same weight, not once or twice, but time and time again?

When marketers promote these products, they are not selling you the product or service as much as they are selling you the illusion of what your life might be like *if* you were successful in losing the 15 or 20 pounds you've been carrying around for months or years. In fact, the product often has less to do with your decision to purchase it than it does how it is presented to you.

Have you ever seen a commercial for a weight-loss product or program with a bunch of unhappy, sweaty overweight people struggling while exercising, or sitting around a table eating meal-replacement bars, drinking caffeinated weight-loss shakes, or choking down another bland salad with a piece of dry chicken on top, with the words, "This product is Guaranteed to help you lose weight when combined with a healthy diet, and exercise?"

It's not likely you have, or ever will, because that sends the wrong message. And that message is what is true: weight loss and dieting is a struggle the way we do it, and inviting struggle into our lives is not a great motivator.

Instead, we see commercials showing groups of "After's." Vibrant, healthy young adults, enjoying themselves in different ideal settings. They may be enjoying a glass of wine at the beach during twilight hours. The tiki torches are burning behind them as they chat with friends, enjoying each other's company in a happy, energetic setting. You often see a plate of food quickly pass in front of the screen just long enough to attract your attention, suggesting this is something you can eat while using this product or program. But it's not food you would normally associate with dieting; it's part of the illusion, and it's so tempting you almost want to reach into the television and grab a bite for yourself.

This is the illusion we buy into. After all, who wouldn't want a little youthful exuberance in his or her life? To feel youthful, energetic, and happy, and maybe add an element of romance. We all know what we're seeing is far from reality, but we buy into the possibility of *what might be* if we were to use whatever product is being advertised.

It's not that the advertisers, or the companies that hire them are being deceitful. Their products will help you lose weight to one degree or another, but the statistics don't lie. The likelihood that you will experience lasting results, or your life will somehow magically transform from the reality it is today to the illusion portrayed by these commercials is infinitesimally small.

One of the more disturbing trends in advertising today is the attempt to make everything appear healthy or healthier. The health and fitness industry has taken off over the past few decades, and everyone wants to capitalize on it, including many companies selling fast, convenience, and snack foods. Some companies advertising what the majority in the healthcare field would consider less than healthy foods now emphasize how much protein or fiber you are getting by consuming their products. They just omit mention of the calories, fats, sugars, and carb content, leading consumers to believe it's a healthy choice because it has 6 grams of protein.

Other convenience-food companies take what are known to be generally unhealthy, empty calorie foods and portray them as healthier choices because they removed the cheese, or mayo, and or replaced an unhealthy snack with a 'healthier' one. This might make the meal less unhealthy, but it doesn't necessarily mean the meal is healthy or nutritious. Understand, they aren't making claims that the meals are healthy; they're simply manipulating the message, which can confuse consumers who might believe it is a healthy choice.

There's a breakfast sandwich I call a "heart attack on a roll." Three eggs, bacon, sausage, ham, and cheese on a roll. Now, if you ate one every morning for breakfast, and we took away the ham or cheese, the sandwich would be less unhealthy – but would it be healthy?

Of the many tools marketers use, one of the most influential is called, "affective conditioning." This is where the product or service being offered is surrounded by things that you, the consumer, already feels good about or wants in your life. An example of how well this tool works to influence your decision to buy a product was shown in a simple study.[69] Two groups of consumers were offered the choice of two pens. Prior to the study, they were told which of the two was the better pen and why, and they were instructed to pick the best-quality pen once they had finished watching a string of advertisements for the pens.

The first group was exposed to repetitive advertisements in which both pens had to stand on their own merits. Their look and perceived quality were the only distinguishing factors describing the pens. When told to select the best pen, the consumers naturally selected the pen they were told was best. The second group was shown the same advertisements with one exception. The advertisements showing the pen of lessor quality used affective conditioning to program or condition the consumers. The lessor quality pen was surrounded with visual and audio cues that are known to make people feel good. It could be anything: puppies, kittens, bunnies, or an activity, or event that everyone generally perceives, or has had a positive experience with, or would feel good having, like signing the paperwork for your brand-new car or home.

You would think that being told in advance which pen was a better-quality writing implement would make people choose it over the lessor pen, and it did for the first group. However, the consumers in the second group, who were conditioned to associate the lessor quality pen with things that made them happy, despite knowing the other pen was a better-quality product, selected the lessor quality pen 70 to 80% of the time.

The point is that we learn through repetition, experience, observation, and exposure to information in our environment. And the advertising we are exposed to becomes a part of the information the brain uses to influence our thoughts, decisions, and actions.

Remember, our brains process billions of bits of information per second, including information gathered through the body's senses. We are only capable of being aware of a fraction of this information,[70] less than one-half of a billionth of a percent, which leaves plenty of room for other information to get into our heads and find a comfortable place to live until it is called upon to influence our thoughts, decisions, and actions.

Oddly enough, as amazing as the subconscious mind is, it does not distinguish between what's real, fantasy, or imaginary.[71] It simply stores the information, processes it, and decides whether to bring it to active thought and conscious awareness, or to hold that information in long-term memory for use at a later time. For example, we all know dieting is as much fun as having a root canal; it just lasts longer. But when you see commercial after commercial of happy, healthy young adults enjoying themselves in a variety of positive social situations, drinking wine, and passing a plate of food between them that would wipe out a day's calorie count, you begin to associate what you know to be a less than pleasurable experience with the illusion of something other than what it really is.

Your mind, affectively conditioned, will lead you in the direction of using a product or service that you associate with happiness, whether or not using this product, plan, or service is the most efficient way for you to achieve your weight-loss goals.

Chapter Summary

- The physical barriers to successful weight loss and maintenance have to do with effects that time, age, dieting, diet, and exposure to chemicals, pollutants, and toxins have on the body's ability to efficiently process and assimilate the foods we consume.

- The genetic barriers have less to do with the genes giving us the characteristics that make us the unique individuals we are and more to do with the fat genes FTO, IRX3, and IRX5.

- The fat genes have an on/off switch that can be controlled by adding polyphenol-rich foods to your diet while minimizing the dietary intake of foods known to raise blood sugar levels.

- The psychological barriers are the most difficult to address because they involve changing deeply ingrained beliefs, paradigms, and behaviors.

- The environmental barriers include all things in our environment that affect our ability to lose excess weight and maintain a healthier weight and waistline.

- Measures taken to protect our food sources negatively affect the body's ability to efficiently process and assimilate the foods we consume into fat-burning energy.

- Affective conditioning is the programming of consumers' minds to associate a particular product or service with something that already makes them feel good.

- The quality of a product or service offered in advertisements often has less to do with the decision to buy than with the feel-good imagery used to promote it.

A Cure 4 Dieting

Part II

7

Weight Loss Is Not the Ultimate Goal

Up to this point, this book has been impressing upon you the idea that weight gain is a symptom of more than just overeating; and as such, weight gain is not a problem that can be addressed by using traditional weight-loss and dieting practices alone.

How can we expect to manage and control our weight when the only options available to help us do so are both the cure and the cause of weight gain? It's the *dieter's dilemma*: a self-perpetuating cycle of weight loss, weight gain, and unsustainable dieting practices.

It's not that dieting doesn't work. It's just that it doesn't work well the way we usually do it. When I set out to learn why I was gaining weight after each of the many diets I employed, the goal wasn't to find a better way to lose weight, much less to discover a way to improve and accelerate the results of my weight-loss efforts. That was just an added bonus. My interests were in finding out *why* I couldn't keep the weight off once I had lost it, and why I gained more weight back than I had ever lost while dieting.

I assumed that, because my injury and surgery had left me sedentary and unable to exercise, I was destined to have some weight issues – but not to the degree I was dealing with at the time. What I couldn't understand was why I gained over 40 pounds during the five years I was dieting, especially when I was watching what I was eating and I continued to moderate my post-diet intake, often eating just one or two meals per day.

I remember starting to think it was me, that maybe I was genetically predisposed to being overweight. But little did I know that I would soon come across the reasons why dieters struggle to maintain their hard-earned results. And I would later find a way to easily address those reasons, solving a problem that has plagued dieters for the better part of a century.

Outside of certain medical conditions, the general assumption has been that weight gain is purely the result of overeating and/or inactivity. As a result, restricting caloric intake and increasing energy expenditure have been the primary focus of the majority of weight-loss and dieting strategies. This approach to weight loss is prescribed by over one million health-care professionals and affiliates in the United States alone,[1] and has become the global standard.

What was Einstein's definition of insanity? "Insanity is doing the same thing over, and over, but expecting different results." If so, then we all must be a little bit crazy, because the average American dieter will make as many as four to five attempts each year to lose weight. That's twice the number of attempts made by our friends across the pond, in the UK[2] and Europe. But the question is: How many diets will it take before you realize that something is wrong with your weight-loss strategy? More important, how much of your life are you willing to sacrifice for dieting?

Sacrifice Is a Strong Word

Sacrifice is a strong word, but if you were to consider all you have to give up and all you have to deal with while dieting, you have to admit you are sacrificing a lot for temporary results. It's not just giving up your favorite foods, or suffering the constant hunger, relentless cravings, low energy levels, and expense that come with dieting; it's also the physical and mental stresses associated with dieting; the compromises we make in our family and social life; the anxiety and mood swings that are the result of low blood sugar; the depletion of vital nutrients; and the reduced levels of the feel-good hormone serotonin.[3]

It's the agitation, irritability, and even depression associated with the production and secretion of cortisol in response to low glucose levels, and the frustration that comes with watching weeks and months of hard-earned results reverse themselves once your diet comes to an end. But the heaviest price we pay is the most disturbing of all: the negative effects that cyclical dieting has on our physical health and wellbeing.[4]

If you were to guess how much time you think the average dieter spends dieting over the course of a lifetime, what would your guess be? Would it add up to two years? Four or maybe five years? According to one research study, the average female dieter will spend not two, four, or even five years dieting, but an incredible seventeen years of her life dieting.[5] That's an average of 204 months, or 6,205 days, or 148,920 hours. Other studies reveal the average female dieter will spend six months of every year dieting in one form or another, and will do so for an estimated thirty-one years of her life, whereas the average male dieter will spend twenty-eight years attempting to improve upon his weight and physical appearance.[6]

If you allow eight hours per day for sleep, you can expect to spend just shy of 100,000 hours of your precious life restricting caloric intake; watching everything you eat and avoiding the foods you enjoy most; and dealing with the frustration, constant hunger, cravings, stress, moodiness, and expense of dieting. That's a heavy price to pay for temporary results, don't you think?

The sad part is that the other half of the time when we're not dieting we are beating ourselves up for not being able to keep the weight off. One body-image survey revealed that 97% of women have negative body-image thoughts about themselves daily.[7] Some of the survey takers admit to upwards of 50 to 100 negative body-image thoughts per day, and it's not just noticing that they could lose a little weight; some comments reported by participants are downright self-abusive.

Think about the incredible advancements we have made in everything from agriculture to technology over the past century; inventors, innovators, and entrepreneurs have improved the performance, functionality, and effectiveness of most everything we use to make life a little easier. But despite the advancements in nutritional science, the results achieved through our weight-loss efforts have remained relatively unchanged, with the vast majority of dieters failing to achieve the long-term weight-loss success they desire and deserve.

It's Time for Change!

When I first applied what I had learned to my weight-loss efforts, it went against all I believed to be true about weight loss and dieting. Not only did I eat more and more often, I found I had to remind myself to eat something throughout the day, and on occasion actually had to push myself to eat something. This was very strange because my "programming" told me I was supposed to be hungry when dieting, and if I wasn't hungry when dieting, I wasn't losing any weight.

That was my preconceived notion about losing weight, which quickly changed when I realized the extraordinary results that came with addressing the barriers, blocks, and changes – what I call the BBCs – influencing my weight-loss efforts.

In multiple trials, dieters exceeded their weight-loss expectations. My personal average was just over 10 pounds lost in the first week alone, with a record of just over 12 pounds lost in one seven-day period. In the weeks to follow, my weight loss was double what I had experienced with dieting alone, and all I was doing was eating real food in a way that allowed my body to efficiently process and assimilate the food I was consuming.

It's been over three years since my final trials, and my focus has long since changed from weight loss and dieting to stabilization and maintenance. I'm still testing the waters to see what I can get away with, but having addressed the barriers, blocks, and changes, my weight-loss and management struggles are over. I now have the freedom to eat what I want, when I want, and I never have to worry about my waistline or permanent weight gain – ever again.

Understanding how the foods I consume affect my body has allowed me to manage my weight more efficiently than I ever could have done with dieting alone. I'd like nothing more than for you to have the same freedom. I call this "optimization." And optimization can be adapted to most any weight-loss strategy. Your approach to optimization, weight loss, and stabilization starts with addressing the pitfalls of weight control: restriction, sustainability, transitioning, and maintenance.

Restriction

Each of us has a different tolerance for dieting and for restricting our caloric intake. If you attempt to follow a strategy that over-restricts caloric intake, has you skipping meals, has you cutting out all sugars, carbs, and fat from your diet for extended periods of time, you will find your weight-loss and maintenance efforts to be grueling, and likely short lived.

It's important to remember that the body perceives weight loss as a potentially dangerous situation, even in today's day and age, and will act to conserve energy to prevent further fat loss, while simultaneously triggering protective mechanisms to store fat and minimize its release. The body wants that fat in order to rebuild vital energy reserves stored in fat, which were and are being lost as a result of your weight-loss efforts. The key to addressing the effects that caloric restriction has on your weight-management efforts is to convince your body that nothing has changed. What I mean by this is, your body will have adapted to a certain dietary intake.

More Meals, More Often

As explained in Part I, if you normally consume three or four full meals and/or snacks per day, and you cut that down to two calorically restrictive meals per day or minimize your caloric intake during those meals, your body will sense this change through the fluctuation of appetite-controlling hormones like leptin, ghrelin, and other chemical messengers signaling the brain that your caloric intake has dropped. So, in optimization, instead of cutting down on meals and snacks, you increase them. Up from two or three to five, six, or seven healthy meals and snacks per day. These are meals and snacks that provide satiating proteins, complex carbs, and healthy fats.

This change will help your weight-loss and management efforts in a few ways. First, feeding yourself regularly throughout the day before the stomach empties will keep the stomach lining partially stretched, or distended, which helps to prevent or minimize the secretion of the hunger hormone ghrelin, thereby limiting the hunger and cravings you would normally feel when dieting.

Second, eating this way will decrease the likelihood of your over-indulging during meals and snacks because you stomach has not fully emptied – you simply won't be all that eager to eat a lot.

Finally, the body will not readily detect a decrease in caloric intake because it is getting a steady stream of calories and nutrients from proteins, complex carbs, and healthy fats. This will prevent large fluctuations in the hormones and chemical messengers that tell the brain to stimulate hunger and cravings.

It's the best of both worlds: eat more often, minimizing the constant hunger and cravings normally experienced when dieting, while you lose or maintain your weight.

Now, there is a method to this that will boost the sustainability factor of your weight-loss and stabilization efforts. The meals and snacks you consume should satisfy your cravings for sweet, sour, and salty, as well as provide an ample supply of healthy fat, protein, complex carbs, and fiber. These foods are slower digesting and require more time and energy to digest, which means you feel fuller longer and burn more calories digesting them in the process. Plus, the fiber slows the release of natural sugars into your system, providing the body with a steady stream of usable energy while minimizing spikes in sugar and preventing large fluctuations in energy levels.

Of course, if an empty stomach were the only thing that triggers hunger and cravings, we'd be done here. But there are other equally important things to consider.

As you may recall from earlier chapters, leptin, or the starvation hormone, is produced by the body's fat cells. And when we begin to lose weight, circulating levels of leptin drop, which signal the brain to stimulate hunger and cravings in an attempt to get you to eat more and thereby elevate the circulating levels of leptin. Leptin is one of a group of hormones produced by fat cells that interacts with other parts of the body, including the brain and liver. Its job is to regulate body weight and maintain it within a relatively narrow range. It works more to moderate long-term food intake and fat storage, and it does this by blocking hunger.

You might see how this effects your weight-loss and maintenance efforts. You want to lose fat and keep it off, but the fat you are losing produces the hormone that blocks hunger, which means the more fat you lose, the less hunger-blocking leptin is being produced and the hungrier you get. The good news is that leptin is only one of many chemicals and hormones regulating appetite, and the effects of decreasing leptin levels associated with weight loss can be addressed in a number of ways.

First, you can start by replacing unhealthy saturated fats, or fats that are solid at room temperature, like butter, cream, full-fat milk, and cheese, as well as the fats found in non-grass-fed beef and pork, processed deli meats, sausages, salami, and skin on chicken. You exchange those for healthier polyunsaturated and monounsaturated fats that can be found in fatty fish, avocados, nuts, seeds, olive oil, dark chocolate, whole eggs, and certain cheeses which, although high in saturated fatty acids, can help raise good cholesterol levels (HDL) in certain circumstances.[8] The body's response to consuming healthy fats while dieting is the release of a hormone called adiponectin from your adipose, or fat tissue, which helps to break down and metabolize fats faster. And because you are consuming healthier fats that are more easily converted into the brown fat the body uses for energy, the body is less likely to stimulate your appetite.

Another way to address falling levels of leptin and the secretion of the hunger hormone is to consume meals and snacks in timed intervals throughout the day. As an early riser, I often consumed six, sometimes seven meals and snacks per day. I enjoyed full-size meals and smaller snacks, and I found on occasion I had to push myself to eat something, which is important for losing weight, not for maintaining it. Eating as much, and as often as I do did challenge my beliefs and all I thought I knew about weight loss and dieting, but the weight kept pouring off.

Moderating Your Favorites

The next restriction you will want to address is the elimination of the foods you enjoy most from your weight-loss efforts. One of the most difficult things to do when dieting is to give up your favorite foods for extended periods of time.

We grow attached to our favorite foods – so much so that researchers are suggesting when we consume certain foods the body releases feel-good chemicals, or endorphins like dopamine, which may in part be responsible for the addictive quality of some of our favorite foods. And that's what makes giving them up a hard thing to do.

Giving up your favorite foods even short term is a challenge for many. Understandably, few people are capable of or willing to eliminate them, or to radically alter their dietary intake permanently for the sake of losing a few pounds and inches – and who could blame them? This is one of reasons why so few dieters ever achieve lasting results.

For some dieters, the answer to minimizing the effects or withdrawals we experience as a result of separating ourselves from our favorite foods is to have a "cheat day" once per week. The concept of a cheat day is not new, and has been successfully used by many to satisfy the cravings associated with dieting, allowing them to continue with their weight-loss efforts a bit longer. However, this method is not for everyone.

Cheat days' work well for those who use the day to enjoy small amounts of their favorite foods sensibly; those lacking self-control can easily overdo it, however, and wipe out the hard-earned results achieved over the prior days and weeks. It can also stall the progress, bringing your efforts to a crawl.

Those lacking self-control during the weight-loss process might wish to avoid the cheat days and focus on healthier versions of their favorite foods that can satisfy the palate on a regular basis. By doing this, they are less likely to go overboard on indulgences when and if they elect to celebrate their success once a week with a favorite meal.

Taking a sensible approach to what and how much you restrict from your caloric intake, and understanding how the foods you consume can either help or hurt your weight-loss efforts will help you to address the restrictions of dieting and avoid that pitfall.

Sustainability

We've all been there. A few weeks or months into our diets, we've lost some weight, or maybe even achieved our weight-loss goals, and we're feeling pretty good about ourselves. And then something catches our attention. Maybe it's the unmistakable scent of barbecue favorites on a neighbor's grill or the smell of freshly baked bread, cookies, or pastries as you pass your favorite bakery.

It could be something as simple as one of those late-night commercials taunting you with sizzling plates of your favorite foods piled high, and you begin to think, *I'm doing good. The weight is coming off; maybe I'll just have one* (insert your favorite weakness here).

The telltale sign is the phrase, "maybe I'll just have one," which marks the beginning of the end of your efforts. You might act on your sensory-induced cravings in the moment, or the very next day. You might even be able to hold off a while longer, but the wheels are in motion. Your senses are heightened. You're tuned into the advertisements that seem to be popping up everywhere, and it's only a matter of time before you stop thinking about it and take that first bite. After all, it can't hurt; it's only just this once.

This is a problem all dieters must contend with, and have for the better part of a century. It doesn't really matter what gets you first – a cookie, brownie, bag of chips, pizza, cheesecake, or something else. It could be a bite of a friend's cheeseburger and a few fries. Oh – better wash that down with an ice cold…?

One bite leads to two, two to three, and before you know it, you find yourself back in your pre-diet routine eating the same foods, in the same way that were responsible for your weight circumstance – and with a slower metabolism to boot. Your diet goes out the window, taking your dreams of maintaining your hard-earned results with it.

Believe it or not, it's not your fault, although you will blame yourself for not having the willpower to stay the course. Never would you think one bite of something would lead to the demise of your weight-loss efforts. Nor would you have ever considered your approach to weight loss might be part of the reason you are unable to sustain your efforts. But the reality of it is that, when you diet, restrict your caloric intake and remove your ability to satisfy what you crave, one bite is all it takes.

I followed the standard weight-loss and dieting strategies to the letter, and I lost weight just like you and every other dieter would – and then I gained all the weight back, and more, just like every other dieter does. Worse still, dieting was sucking the enjoyment out of life. Half the time I was starving myself and the other half I was frustrated, watching the pounds pile back on. I had one thing working in my favor. Ever since I was a kid, I had a penchant for improving things. I always felt that there's always room for improvement. There's a better, more efficient way to do everything, especially if it's something I don't like doing. Toward the end of my "five years of dieting hell," as I like to call it, I learned that when it comes to weight loss and dieting, knowing, not following, is the key to success.

Lasting weight loss and management success requires three things:

• A sustainable strategy to help you reach your goal.

• A well-executed exit strategy for transitioning to normal life.

• A maintenance strategy that allows you to efficiently manage your weight *while enjoying all foods sensibly.*

Turning unsustainable weight-loss and dieting strategies into sustainable weight-loss and dieting strategies is as simple as eliminating, addressing, or improving those things about dieting that you find most undesirable. To address the sustainability issues in your weight-loss efforts, write down everything about dieting you don't like. Break it down into categories, if you like, such as:

- What I can deal with.
- What I struggle with.
- What I find unbearable about weight loss and dieting.

If you find the constant hunger and cravings associated with dieting are the worst, deal with them by increasing your meal intervals, consuming satiating foods, and including healthier versions of your favorite foods. You might add a couple of calories, but it'll help you minimize the cravings and allow you to stay in the game long enough to reach your weight-loss goals.

Also, increase your ingestion of healthy fats and minimize the saturated fats. You'll also want to be sure to satisfy your taste for sweet and salty, as well as your taste for bitter and sour, if you are so inclined. You can also optimize the efficiency of your body's digestive process by making a few simple dietary changes, which I'll share with you in the next chapter.

Learn what your specific barriers, blocks, and changes are and address them. Avoid mixing carbs with animal proteins. Use and consume products that help support a healthy gut biome – fiber, probiotics, and other prebiotics. Include an abundance of polyphenol-rich fruits and veggies to assist in the conversion of white fat into the brown fat we use for energy and heat.

If moodiness, agitation, and frustration while dieting is one of your peeves, learn to satisfy your cravings with healthier versions of your favorite foods. This will help minimize the emotional effects of dieting and the falling levels of serotonin, the happy hormone. In the worst-case scenario, incorporate a small amount of a favorite treat to take the edge off, but don't do it every day, or twice a day, and follow the rules given in the next chapter to minimize the effects these foods might have on your weight-loss efforts.

If you find your family and social life difficult to deal with when dieting, use a weight-loss strategy that allows you to consume real foods that can be shared or consumed with family and friends or ordered when dining out. Avoid over-restrictive, liquid, or single-food weight-loss strategies, and other diets in which you cannot consume whole foods with your family and friends at mealtime.

Remember, once you reach your target weight and have optimized your system, nothing is off the table as long as you follow a few simple rules. You will be surprised how this simple detail will help to support the sustainability of your weight-loss and management efforts.

Transitioning and Stabilization

The next goal in your weight-loss efforts is to transition out of your weight-loss strategy and to stabilize your post-diet weight. It sounds easy enough, but post-diet weight gain is the wall you, me, and every other dieter on the planet runs into when the diet comes to an end – unless we're willing to continue the restrictions and compromises of the weight-loss strategy we've employed. That's an option few dieters have any interest in.

Transitioning is the most crucial aspect of your weight-management efforts, and yet few dieters have ever heard of it, much less understand the important role it plays in helping to stabilize a healthier weight and waistline. You might believe that dieting itself is the most important part of weight management, and if you are only looking to "rent" your results for a short while, you'd be right. But if you want to own your weight-loss results, you need a *sustainable exit strategy*.

Anyone can lose weight, but keeping it off has been a problem for dieters ever since dieting for aesthetic reasons was popularized over a century ago. Consider the stats. Depending on which source you cite, upwards of 95 to 99% of dieters fail to maintain their post-diet weight.

That's because transitioning is the point in time when you begin to migrate back to your pre-diet routine and reintroduce some of your favorite foods. It also marks the point when you stop losing weight, and start gaining weight which happens as you know, for two main reasons.

The first reason is that your body has adapted to a decrease in caloric intake by slowing your metabolism. How much the metabolism slows depends on a number of different factors; however, it can slow by up to 24% over twelve weeks of dieting. When your diet comes to an end, and you begin to reintroduce foods higher in fat, carbs, and sugar content, you also increase the number of calories above what your body is capable of efficiently burning with its slower metabolism, which for dieters means weight gain. The second reason is that the body is programmed to store fat, not to release it. As explained in Part I, it perceives fat loss as a loss of vital energy reserves stored in fat, and will work to rebuild those reserves, which is more easily accomplished when your caloric intake goes unopposed by dietary restrictions.

Abrupt Transitioning

It used to be there were only two ways to exit a diet. The first, more common among first timers and inexperienced dieters, was to immediately revert to their pre-diet dietary habits. But abrupt transitioning from a weight-loss and dieting strategy back to your pre-diet lifestyle is by far the least effective way to stabilize a healthier weight and waistline. Indeed, this approach puts most dieters on the fast track to post-diet weight gain (PDWG) and another round of dieting, even if you are moderating your caloric intake.

It's only normal that, after weeks or months of starving yourself and avoiding the foods you most enjoy, to sink your teeth into your favorite foods. But suddenly dumping any amount of unhealthy fats, carbs, grease, and sugars, or in the case of processed foods, large quantities of salt, preservatives, colorings, and chemical stabilizers, into a digestive system ill-prepared to handle these foods, will not only lead to PDWG but also cause varying degrees of gastric distress, and the need to remove yourself from polite society.

Take my advice on this. Your body requires time to accommodate itself to these foods. If you are going to reintroduce them, they should be added slowly and in limited quantities. Painful cramping, bloating, gas, and the sudden urgency to explosively evacuate your bowels is no way to celebrate your weight-loss success.

Gradual Transitioning

The second exit strategy, which is less abrupt and is the approach used by experienced dieters, is to gradually reintroduce one's favorite foods. Gradual transitioning affords the body the opportunity to slowly adjust to an increase in caloric intake, and offers the chance to satisfy cravings at a measured pace while controlling the intake of unhealthy fats, carbs, sugar, and processed foods.

This approach also provides an opportunity to monitor how these foods affect your body, which is one of the keys to stabilizing and maintaining a healthier weight and waistline. Once you understand how the foods you are consuming affect your body, you can modify your consumption of them and minimize the negative influence they have on your weight-management efforts.

Experienced dieters transition gradually to help slow and or minimize PDWG, but what they don't realize is just how close they are to stabilizing their weight in the long term. This is where knowing how to enjoy all foods sensibly comes in handy.

Gradual transitioning will serve you best if you're weight-loss strategy includes the consumption of whole foods, or a combination of whole and prepackaged foods. It will not prevent post-diet weight gain. It will only slow its progress because, without addressing the barriers, blocks, and changes, or BBCs, your body will continue to process the foods you consume inefficiently, and will continue its efforts to restore the fat lost while dieting.

New Generation Transitioning

If you are mid-diet or are nearing the end of a diet, this third option is your best bet for stabilizing a healthier weight and waistline. It combines gradual transitioning from a weight-loss strategy with some or all of the information contained in the next chapter.

If done purposefully, it will improve your ability to stabilize and maintain a healthier weight. This third option minimizes PDWG because you have yet to address the BBCs influencing your weight as a whole. As you now address the barriers, blocks, and changes as described in Chapter 6, while transitioning, your weight will stabilize and you may likely find yourself losing more weight, which was my experience when this method was first used.

If your approach to weight loss involved restricting your caloric intake, consuming mostly whole foods, but did not include addressing the BBCs, this option is by far your best bet at minimizing PDWG. However, if your weight-loss strategy was along the lines of a ketogenic or prepackaged food diet, be aware that you are likely to add more weight when your diet comes to an end. With both of these food specific type diets, the body requires more time to adjust to the increase in caloric intake from the variety of whole foods being reintroduced to your dietary intake.

Progressive Transitioning

The fourth option is the most effective option, by far. When it comes to weight loss and dieting, I believe we are all a bit impatient. The process is tedious, frustrating, and requires lengthy periods of restriction and compromise – which are just a few of many issues making dieting a less than pleasurable experience. Not to mention that most diets are rather generic and do not cater to the specific tastes and needs of the dieter. They leave us hungry, stressed, moody, and craving foods sure to wipe out your daily calorie count. Foods which once tasted great can bring an untimely end to any diet.

Traditionally, the diets we employ have a beginning and an end. The day our diets start, we cut calories and eliminate the foods we believe are responsible for weight gain and we begin to consume only those foods we believe will help us achieve our weight-loss goals. In the process, we suffer ourselves to consume the same bland unsatisfying foods day in and day out until we reach our target weight, or until we can no longer tolerate the restrictions.

Now, imagine for a moment, learning to permanently improve your body's ability to efficiently process and assimilate the foods you consume, transforming them into the essential nutrients and fat-burning energy required to function optimally. You do this by making a few simple changes in how you eat along with small behavioral changes described in Chapter 6. This fourth strategy was developed specifically to accelerate the results achieved through dieting for those of us without the time, desire, or ability to exercise. I fell into the latter category. Little did I know how well it would work to improve and accelerate the results of my dieting efforts.

This option focuses on improving your ability to optimally digest the foods you consume. It works equally well on women and men, despite the slight anatomical differences between the male and female digestive tracts. That's because it's not as much a diet as it is a tune-up for your digestive system. It offers an effective solution for improving overall health and function of the digestive system, and it provides an efficient means for managing your weight without radical dietary changes or heavy restrictions.

The key to option four is transitioning without transitioning, which may sound a bit confusing, but is easily accomplished by incorporating the transition into the weight-loss strategy itself while you simultaneously identify and address the BBCs that are interfering with your ability to lose, stabilize, and maintain a healthier weight.

Progressive transitioning is part and parcel of your weight-loss and dieting strategy, using whole foods as the primary source of your caloric intake. I'll spare you the complex details of exactly how it all works. Suffice to say, option four will help you lose and maintain a healthier weight and waistline. You develop a healthy weight-loss momentum and achieve your target weight faster while ensuring sustainability.

This succeeds because you gradually add some of your favorite foods or their healthier versions along the way. This helps to minimize the cravings and calms the separation anxiety many dieters experience when eliminating their favorite foods for extended periods of time, and it virtually eliminates the sustainability issues that arise from the hunger associated with more traditional weight-loss and dieting strategies.

The goal here is to acquire the knowledge and skills to successfully stabilize and maintain your weight. You break the vicious cycle of weight loss, weight gain, and dieting, and optimize your body's ability to process the foods you consume into fat-burning energy. All the while, this can be accomplished with nothing more than enjoying real whole foods with friends and family, which is another benefit of this approach; it eliminates the social awkwardness that comes with customary dieting. Instead of being an outsider and eating unpalatable foods no one else wants to eat, you'll be sharing real food everyone can enjoy together.

By making a few dietary changes, you can crank up the heat on your body's fat-burning machine; minimize the effects of leptin, ghrelin, an unhealthy gut biome, and the body's survival programming; and flip your fat-storing switch to off. And once you've reached your goal, nothing is off the table because you will have formed healthy and effective weight-sustaining habits. In fact, you can enjoy all foods sensibly without worrying about your waistline or permanent weight gain because you will know how to efficiently manage your weight.

Chapter 8 presents what I believe are some of the most effective strategies for improving your ability to lose pounds and to stabilize at a healthier weight, with or without exercise. As I tested this information, I discovered that the more strategies I incorporated into my weight loss and management efforts, the faster the weight came off and the easier it was to maintain my results while enjoying my favorite foods sensibly. Isn't this what all dieters have wanted all along?

Some Personality Types

We are all little different and as individuals we approach the various aspects of life in different ways. Some of these ways can become obstacles for successful weight loss and stabilization strategies or can be ability-enhancers. Are you any of these people?

Micro-Managers

Micro-managers generally take their weight and appearance very seriously. They tend to be a bit obsessive, even self-critical about themselves, and will examine their appearance every chance they get to determine if and what part of their body may need some work. And they usually find something they are not happy with.

This approach tends to be a bit tedious and can lead to increased levels of stress and frustration, mostly because body weight can easily fluctuate between 1 to 5 pounds daily, depending on any number of factors including, but not limited to, hydration, salt consumption, specific types of foods consumed, and the frequency at which urine is eliminated or bowels evacuated.

Although, micro-managing may help you maintain your weight, the added stress and frustration associated with it may not be worth the effort. It can lead to unhealthy eating behaviors and secretion of the stress hormone, cortisol, which is public enemy number one for your weight management efforts.

Nine to Fivers

Nine to fivers treat weight management much like a job. They typically restrict caloric intake and avoid the foods they believe responsible for adding unwanted pounds and inches for four or five days of the week, and allow themselves free rein to enjoy their favorites the other two or three days of the week.

This method works fairly well, provided you don't overdo it on your off days and have the willpower to pick up where you left off every Monday morning for as long as you want to keep the weight off.

Although this approach does work for some, the off days can become all the days, which brings you back to square one: finding another diet. In addition, this strategy can wreak havoc on the gastrointestinal system, depending on the dietary indulgences during off days.

Optimizers

Optimizers adopt healthier (not obsessive) eating behaviors and enjoy their favorite foods sensibly. They are generally aware of how the foods they consume affect their bodies, and they attempt to avoid consuming large quantities of foods that negatively affect their weight on a daily basis. They incorporate one or more of the strategies described in this text to optimize their ability to efficiently process and assimilate the foods they consume into fat-burning energy, which allows them some leeway on the indulgence side of things.

Optimizers watch their weight, but do not obsess about it. They understand how the foods they consume affect the body and know that consuming an abundance of carbs or sugar-rich foods during a meal, over the course of a weekend, on the holidays, or while on vacation will cause water retention, dietary bloating, and weight gain. But they do not stress when they see a few extra few pounds on the scale because they know how to quickly eliminate them.

Chapter Summary

- Weight loss is not the ultimate goal.

- Dieting works – just not the way we do it.

- The average dieter sacrifices 17 years, 6,205 days, or 148,920 hours of their precious life dealing with the constant hunger, cravings, and expense of dieting.

- Restricting caloric intake triggers protective mechanisms in the body to store fat, not to release it.

- Simple changes to your dietary habits can minimize the effects that restricting caloric intake has on the body.

- If you have to do something you don't enjoy, learn to do it right the first time and avoid having to repeat the process.

- A successful weight loss strategy requires three things:

  – A sustainable weight-loss and dieting strategy.

  – A well-executed exit strategy for transitioning to normal life.

  – A maintenance strategy for efficiently managing your weight *while enjoying all foods sensibly*.

- Transitioning is the most crucial aspect of a weight-loss and dieting strategy.

- The ability to stabilize and maintain a healthier weight and waistline has eluded dieters for the better part of a century – it's time for a change.

- Whether losing weight or maintaining it, the foods you consume should be nothing less than delicious and satisfying.

- It's time to stop "renting" your results and take ownership of your body!

8

The Do's and Don'ts of Dieting

This is worth repeating: If you have to do something you don't like doing, learn to do it right the first time; this way, you only have to do it once. Next time should be reserved for the pleasures and necessities in life, and dieting is neither – life is too short to diet more than once!

Besides, who wants to sacrifice seventeen years[10] of his or her life struggling with the constant hunger, cravings, stress, moodiness, and expense of dieting, which by the very nature of dieting can provide results that are temporary at best? It's not enough to depend on dieting the way we've learned to do it. Progress is taking its toll on the environment, on our food sources, and on our bodies. The playing field has changed, and our bodies have changed, and we must change our approach if we want fast and lasting results.

Having reached this point, you now know that weight gain is not the problem, and it is not solely the result of overeating. *It's a symptom.* It's the result of a combination of factors contributing to the physical changes brought about and accelerated by age, lifestyle, diet, and the physical, genetic, environmental, and psychological barriers influencing our weight circumstance.

To own your hard-earned results and put an end to the vicious cycles of weight loss, weight gain, and dieting, you need to support the singularly focused weight-loss strategies with the knowledge and skills to improve their effectiveness; you do that by addressing all the factors influencing your weight circumstance, rather than just the one. Only then you will be able to effectively control your weight-management efforts.

What Doesn't Work

Over the years, the weight-loss industry has issued its fair share of wonder plans, foods, supplements, strategies, products, and equipment, all promising to transform your life. And although some may have helped some dieters lose weight, there are two things they all have in common: restricted caloric intake, and post-diet weight gain.

The problem is, and always has been, that not all weight-loss strategies work for everyone, and the ones that do work for you only work for as long as you continue them. Once you stop, the weight comes back. And more often than not, it brings its friends and you wind up heavier than when you started, a little more frustrated and confused.

In my efforts to find a sustainable weight-loss strategy, I cycled through different dieting plans. Some were structured toward consumers, but the majority were common do-it-yourself or self-governed plans. And like millions of other dieters, I lost weight using a popular plan, only to have the weight come back with a vengeance. This was despite the fact that I moderated my post-diet intake and I consumed foods I believed to be healthy.

Now, it might be just me, but I found it difficult to justify spending the time, or another thousand plus dollars, to lose the same weight. And I certainly had no interest in paying hundreds of dollars every month for the rest of my life, just to fit into smaller pants. There had to be a better way.

The plans employed over the years included strategies offered by the health-care industry, prepackaged plans, no-carbs, low-carbs, no-fat, low-fat, soy diets, soup diets, all-meat, no-meat, pescatarian, vegetarian, no-sugar diets, water diets, fasting, and what I call single-food diets like the grapefruit and avocado diets that were all the rage then. Although I personally don't care for the thought of changing the body's chemistry, whether doing so with supplements or specific diet plans designed to have that effect, I did dabble in them to see their effectiveness. They were no different in providing lasting results than those achieved through any other weight loss strategy. As a result of those efforts, though, I learned what works, what doesn't, and why.

As you read this chapter, understand that each of us responds in different ways to the weight-loss strategies available to us. You may respond favorably to a particular strategy that others do not, and your body may respond a little differently when consuming certain foods. But the one thing that remains the same, outside of slight anatomical differences in the male and female digest tracts, is this: we digest our foods in the same way, and we all encounter the barriers, blocks, and changes that interfere with our ability to lose weight and keep it off.

The category of "doesn't work" includes approaches that, on their own, do not improve the effectiveness and/or efficiency of your weight-loss efforts. They include *elimination diets*, in which you attempt to eliminate all fats, carbs, sugars, meat, or other designated foods. These may help you to lose weight initially, but they come with above-average difficulty as far as sustainability goes. Eventually, the body reaches a plateau where it accommodates the dietary change, and you stop losing weight.

Single-source diets include soy diets, soup diets, all-meat, liquid diets, juice diets, protein shake diets, water diets, and diets concentrating on items like potatoes, grapefruit, and avocados. These, too, will help you lose weight initially, but not because of any miraculous benefit they provide; rather, the heavily restricted intake triggers post-diet weight gain, and the need to diet again.

Restricting Your Caloric Intake

The most common approach to weight loss is to simply restrict your caloric intake. Although it works for anyone wishing to lose unsightly pounds and inches, on its own it has proven itself to be more the enemy of weight-loss efforts than its ally.

On the one hand, you can't lose weight without restricting calories. On the other hand, it slows the body's metabolism, which makes ongoing weight loss a struggle. That is, the body responds to a decrease in caloric intake by stimulating the desire to feed, which means constant hunger and cravings. Restricting your caloric intake for as little as a few days to a week will trigger protective mechanisms in the body to store fat, not release it. Unfortunately, these mechanisms designed to protect and preserve the body's energy reserves continue to work well beyond the day your diet comes to an end, thereby minimizing the chances of maintaining your hard-earned results.

Single-Style Approaches

Diets that utilize a single food are commonly associated with fad dieting, and are on the top of the "doesn't work" list, if for no other reason than the sustainability factor. The concept of eating one type of "miracle" food every day appears harmless enough, until you read the fine print. That says "When combined with a healthy diet, and exercise… "This in some cases requires you to consume half the calories you would normally consume in a day.

How is that different from anything else you've done in your attempts to lose weight? It's not! You are working just as hard to lose weight by restricting caloric intake, maybe some exercising, and eliminating the foods you enjoy most from your dietary intake. The only difference is that you're adding something extra to your diet that someone says has miraculous weight-loss powers when fed to lab rats. There may indeed be some research showing the miracle food as supporting weight loss, but do your own research. Question everything about it. Where is it from? How does it work? What else do I have to do for it to work, and how will it affect my body?

These are important questions to ask because recent trends have moved toward the marketing of newly discovered miracle foods from far-off places where the indigenous population has a zero-obesity rate. Remember, it's what they *don't* say that is equally if not more important. What may not be mentioned is that the majority of the people who consume that wonder food have never consumed junk food or fast-foods, and they sustain themselves on locally grown produce, fruits, berries, and fish.

There are a number of foods considered to be "super foods," but they are far from miraculous. It's no miracle if you consume the wonder food, or supplements made from them and cut out half the calories from your daily intake. Not to mention, consuming large amounts of one specific food, or having to consume one type of food with each meal, day after day, gets old fast. Many of these diets are extremely restrictive, and may not be the healthiest way to lose weight.

The point is, step back and look at the bigger picture before you jump in. Don't take everything at face value, lest you end up disliking a superfood that can actually benefit your weight loss efforts when consumed sensibly.

Supplements and Gimmicks

Dietary supplements and other chemical-based products are increasingly popular with dieters looking for an edge or an easy way to shed unsightly fat. These products, for the most part, do exactly as they say they do, whether that is to temporarily stimulate the body's metabolism, suppress the appetite, or just boost energy levels for a few hours. But they affect each of us differently. It's not uncommon for those using these products to experience unwanted side effects.

Your tolerance of these products may be higher or lower than the next person's, which is something you need to learn for yourself; but before you do, inquire with friends, family, and co-workers who may have used these types of products. They'll share their experiences and can tell you what to expect. If there are any side effects, like the jitters, restlessness, insomnia, lightheadedness, nausea, dizziness, vomiting, constipation, or other digestive problems, you might reconsider.

For example, many of these products contain high doses of caffeine, which is likely safe for most adults when used sensibly; however, high doses of caffeine over long periods of time can cause insomnia, nervousness and restlessness, stomach irritation, nausea and vomiting, increased heart rate and respiration, and other side effects.[11] Also, ask if they are still taking them, and if not, why and when did they stop? What was the cost, and what happened when they stopped taking them? Did they gain weight or experience any withdrawal symptoms?

If you elect to use weight-loss supplements and other chemicals designed to suppress the appetite or stimulate the metabolism, ask yourself: *How long am I willing to submit my body to the effects of these products, and what they might be doing to my health?*

Artificial Sweeteners

There is some controversy as to the benefits of artificial sweeteners. On the one hand, if you are diabetic or pre-diabetic, artificial sweeteners count as zero on the diabetic scale, but when consumed can cause a spike in insulin levels.[12] On the other hand, artificial sweeteners are reported to cause a decrease in insulin sensitivity and affect the brain by lowering dopamine levels, which causes intense cravings for starches and sugar-rich foods.[13]

Artificial sweeteners are on the "what works versus what doesn't work" fence. If you have blood sugar issues, are pre-diabetic, or are diabetic, t hey may be a necessity. But if you believe your weight-loss efforts will dramatically improve simply by consuming artificially sweetened foods and beverages, don't get your hopes up. Although artificially sweetened products and beverages are low in calories themselves, studies on the effects they have on the body show that consuming them can actually increase caloric intake.[14] Dieters using these products should weigh the benefits, as well as consider the potential adverse effects.

Out with the Old

As dieters, we cannot continue to blindly follow old paradigms, traditions, and practices. As mentioned, one of the most common social habits is eating three square meals per day, and that continues despite decades-old research suggesting that eating this way supports weight gain, and is neither the healthiest nor the most efficient way to provide the body with the nutrients and energy it requires to function at its best.

Questioning everything you do on a regular basis does sound time-consuming, but it takes only a few brief seconds of introspection to see if your habits are controlling your actions, if they fit your life today, if they help or hinder your weight-management efforts. Do they need to be addressed, improved upon, or eliminated? This especially pertains to your eating behaviors.

However, it also applies to how you approach dieting and weight stabilization. If you are among the 1 to 5% of dieters who are successful in losing weight and in keeping it off, and you are happy with living with the restrictions necessary to do so, congratulations! But if you are among the 95 to 99% of dieters not willing to live a life of restriction and compromise, you must question your approach and see what you can do to improve your results, with little or no compromise.

Forming New Habits

One of the challenges facing dieters is the ability to replace old habits, paradigms, and routines with new ones. Many of us have misconceptions about how long it actually takes to change these behaviors. This in part is due to the abundance of misinformation on the topic. New habits can be formed in a few days, however, changing or replacing old behaviors and paradigms requires time – and the amount of time it takes depends on how deeply ingrained the behavior is.[15]

Maxwell Maltz, a plastic surgeon, famous for his book *Psycho-Cybernetics*, stated that it takes twenty-one days for patients who have had facial reconstruction surgery to start getting used to their new look. Unfortunately, this information was taken out of context and used by others to promote their habit-changing agendas, leading to the widespread misconception that it takes only twenty-one days to change a habit – or to change your life.

This twenty-one days seemed very doable for those desiring to improve or change their lives without having to put too much effort into it, and they spent millions on programs that would likely never change anything other than the simplest behaviors. Countless millions believed it possible to turn their lives around in a mere twenty-one days, a myth that lives on fifty years later.

The misconception was laid to rest by Phillip Lally, a health psychology researcher at University College of London, whose 2009 study determined that it took an average of sixty-six days to change a simple habit and have it become second nature. However, Lally also discovered that the more deeply ingrained the behavior, the longer it took to change it. Some habits take upwards of 254 days, or approximately eight and a half months to modify or change.[16]

I'm sure, if you do the math, you'll see why it's difficult for us to change even our most basic eating behaviors. If the average person's diet lasts only five weeks, two days, and forty-three minutes,[17] or just over thirty-seven days, how can we expect to change or replace a deeply ingrained behavior we've practiced 1,095 times a year and 10,950 times for each ten years of life? This certainly explains why it's so easy for us to slip back into our old ways when our diets come to an end.

I'll be the first to admit, the thought of dieting for 254 days sounds far from pleasant, but remember that it's not dieting you're looking to change. The goal is to simply make a few modifications to how you eat so as to improve your body's ability to process and assimilate the foods you consume, turning them into the essential nutrients and energy the body requires to function at optimal levels. Compared to dieting, that's a breeze.

A Commitment to Lose Weight

Every year millions of people make New Year's weight-loss resolutions, but only a few percent will achieve them. Ever wonder why? It may be hard to believe, but weight loss has its seasons, and winter isn't one of them. Winter is the most difficult time of year to lose weight, which is not to say that it can't be done, but attempting to lose weight in winter is like swimming upstream – it can be exhausting.

Winter weight loss goes against the body's natural instincts to preserve itself. To our distant ancestors, winter meant leaner times – a time when food was not always readily available. Fruiting plants, shrubs, and trees were dormant and provided little if any sustenance. Animals migrated away following other food sources, or hibernated, or flew south to winter in warmer weather. And those that remained behind competed for the same food sources as we did.

Because food was often scarce, and the potential for going long periods without adequate sustenance was high, we developed instincts to build fat reserves that would help us through long winters and leaner times. The fat put on in warmer months offered the extra benefit of providing warmth and insulation from the elements, and helped to protect our vital organs.

Another survival mechanism making winter weight loss more difficult is the metabolic changes that occur as a result of our efforts. As you may remember, one of the first things the body does to preserve energy in response to a decrease in caloric intake and weight loss is to slow the metabolism to conserve energy, which means the body is burning less calories, slowing the weight-loss process. The body also limits the energy used to warm the body, which is why we often feel cold when dieting. And feeling cold in wintertime brings most dieters well out of their comfort zone and influences the sustainability of winter weight-loss efforts.

The most important reason, however, has to do not with what the body does to preserve itself. It has to do with how you and your mind perceive resolutions. A *resolution* is nothing more than a decision on what course of action to take, whereas a *commitment* is a pledge, promise, or obligation to do something. To you, it may seem to be nothing more than semantics, but to your mind it makes a big difference!

How many times have you said that you are going to do something, but you never seem to get around to doing it. You may want to go on that vacation, or connect with old friends, or replace a comfortable, broken-down old couch, but until you commit to doing it and set a plan in motion to get it done, it's nothing more than an idea.

Desires without goals are nothing more than dreams.

And goals without action are nothing more than wishful thinking.

The percentage of dieters who achieve lasting results from their weight-loss efforts is the same as the percentage of individuals who succeed in all aspects of life by committing themselves to setting goals and taking action on those goals. Is this a curious coincidence, or something to be considered?

Chapter Summary

- Dieting alone cannot compete with the complexities of weight gain today.

- Restricting your caloric intake without addressing other factors influencing your weight only serves to contribute to your struggles.

- Single-food approaches to weight loss are commonly associated with ineffective fad dieting.

- It's not uncommon to experience unwanted side effects from prolonged use of energy and metabolism boosting supplements.

- Artificial sweeteners can cause increased caloric intake.

- Questioning how and why you do things is the first step toward discovering if outdated paradigms are guiding your decisions and actions.

- The more deeply ingrained a behavior, the longer it takes to change it.

- Stop making resolutions to lose weight, and make a commitment instead.

9

The New Body, Face, and Mind of Weight Loss

Although the intention of this book is to help dieters stabilize their weight and maintain the results of their weight-loss efforts, here you will find principles, tips, and strategies that will not only help you achieve that stabilization and maintain your post-diet weight, but will also contribute to improving and accelerating your weight-loss efforts when purposefully applied to your dieting strategies.

When I first started this journey, it was to find a way to keep the weight off once my dieting had come to an end. Little did I know I would discover the reasons why the majority of dieters' struggle with weight loss, and why dieting on its own is not enough to address the complexities of weight gain. As time passed, the solution became clear on how to maintain the results of my weight-loss efforts; make maintenance part of the weight-loss strategy itself. I never would have imagined that the strategies used to maintain my post-diet weight would also dramatically accelerate and improve the effectiveness of my weight-loss efforts. But they did just that.

There is a popular saying: "There is strength in numbers." This suggests that many people can accomplish more than a single individual. In a way, such is the case with weight loss and dieting. Each of these principles, tips, and strategies will benefit a weight-loss effort and contribute to maintenance success, but cumulatively they can turn up the heat on your fat-burning furnace for even greater results.

Pre- and Probiotics

What's the difference? *Prebiotics* support a healthy balance of the micro-organism, or bacteria, in the gut. *Probiotics* are healthy microorganisms that supplement the gut bacteria and work to benefit digestion.

There are a variety of ways to support the healthy bacteria in the stomach, and employing one or more them will help with your weight-loss and weight-management efforts. Prebiotics can be found in foods like garlic, onions, leeks, asparagus, bananas, cocoa, apples, oats, jicama, and barley. These foods contain a mildly sweet, indigestible polysaccha-ride (complex sugar) that helps support the positive gut bacteria and aids in digestion.

Another way to stimulate the digestive process and support digestion is to drink an 8-ounce glass of water with 1 teaspoon to 1 tablespoon of apple cider vinegar or fresh lemon juice before meals. This helps to sup-port the positive gut bacteria and improves digestion, and when taken just before meals, can reduce caloric intake by filling the stomach.

Probiotics have grown in popularity; and it only took a hundred years for us to catch on to them. In 1907, Nobel Prize winner Elie Metchnikoff, of the Pasteur Institute in Paris, was studying centenarians (people who were living well past 100 years old – In 1907) living in the Caucasus Mountains, a rugged range separating Europe from Southwest Asia. He discovered the health benefits that villagers were deriving from drinking a fermented yogurt beverage similar to kefir, which is a sweetened fermented yogurt beverage you see in stores today. Metchnikoff did not discover the probiotic, *Lactobacillus bulgaricus*, however. That credit goes to Ernst Moro, an Austrian physician who discovered it in 1890. Nevertheless, Metchnikoff identified the benefits derived from it and documented the longevity of the centenarians he was studying.

Today you can't go twenty minutes without seeing a product advertised on television that has been fortified with probiotics. Market shelves are lined with probiotic-enriched products, and every food producer is trying to capitalize on this rise in popularity, presenting probiotics as the key to weight loss and digestive health. However, the occasional addition of probiotics to your dietary intake to promote regularity is not, on its own, enough to address the factors interfering with your ability to lose or maintain a healthier weight.

Should probiotics be incorporated into your diet? Absolutely! They play an important role in optimizing the efficiency of the digestive process. There are trillions of microorganisms in the gut, and as you may recall, the balance of positive, or healthy, gut bacteria keep the negative gut bacteria in check. Probiotics help to support a healthy balance in the gut, which will improve the efficiency of the digestive process. When combined with other strategies, this will optimize your ability to process and assimilate the foods you consume into fat-burning energy.

Probiotics were finally recognized by the World Health Organization (WHO) in 2002 as, "something when given in adequate amounts, confers a benefit to the host."[18] Despite the vague description offered by the WHO, probiotics will help support a healthy gut biome.

As probiotics go, you can find them in pill form, some containing upwards of 10 to 30 billion probiotic microorganisms to well over 1 trillion, the latter are intended to replenish a healthy gut biome in those who are ill and or who are taking long courses of antibiotics. They can also be found in any number of all-natural foods like yogurt, kombucha (tea), sauerkraut, dark chocolate, kimchi (fermented cabbage), miso, green olives, raw cheese,[19] pickles, and many fermented soy products.

You won't have a hard time finding an abundance of probiotic-fortified products like yogurts and kefirs in regular markets, or in health-food stores if you plan on going the organic route. Just be sure the product you're buying is not loaded with sugar, which will negate the benefits of the probiotics. If you don't like plain, unflavored yogurts, try mixing them with flavored yogurts to minimize your sugar intake.

Mixology

The debate rages on as to whether separating animal proteins and carbohydrates in meals is beneficial to your weight-loss and maintenance efforts. Now, to clarify when I say carbohydrates, I am referring to simple carbs found in starchy, sugar-rich foods like white rice, potatoes, pasta, breads, and other wheat, corn, potato, and rice flour-based products, and not the complex carbs found in leafy greens, veggies, oatmeal, beans, lentils, nuts, and seeds.

The body's digestive tract is extremely adaptable, and very capable of digesting both animal proteins and carbs when consumed together – when the digestive tract is 100% healthy. However, when you consider the effects that time, age, lifestyle, diet, personal use of drugs, alcohol, antibiotics, and medications have on the body, as well as our use of and or exposure to chemical-based products, environmental toxins, and pollutants, and the increasing amounts of chemicals, fertilizers, sewerage sludge, pesticides, irradiation, preservatives, artificial sweeteners, flavoring, and food coloring used to grow, protect, and process our foods, plus the chemicals, antibiotics, and hormones used on our animal based food sources, the odds of maintaining the delicate balance of positive and negative gut bacteria , and having a 100% healthy digestive tract, are not in our favor.

Further, it would be foolish to believe that something hasn't changed just because you can't see it, or it hasn't become a big enough problem to be symptomatic. Prevention has been the trend for the past few decades. Preventive measures help minimize the possibility of a particular problem or condition from manifesting, but it is a way also to address subclinical conditions.

For example, when you put on suntan lotion, you are employing a preventive measure to protect yourself from the possibility of getting sunburn or developing skin cancer. When you brush your teeth, you are helping to prevent cavities. When you clean a cut, and apply an antimicrobial ointment, you are protecting against the proliferation of unseen bacteria and microbes that might result in an infection. So, it only makes sense that if some product, service, or strategy has a positive track record in helping with weight management, you would use it to your benefit.

As you apply the strategies shared in this book, you are in effect employing measures to prevent your weight issues from becoming a lifelong problem. In this way, you will find that separating animal proteins and simple carbohydrates as often as possible at mealtime is a benefit for both your weight-management efforts and your lifelong good health.

The concept has been used in weight loss for many years, with positive results despite arguments from the opposition. But much like probiotics, I'm not willing to wait a hundred years to find out who is right and who is wrong. I've employed this optimization strategy, even to an extreme, and in my personal experience, minimizing, or better yet, avoiding, the consumption of animal proteins and simple carbs together especially during the weight loss phase helps improve the effectiveness of weight management!

Separating animal proteins and carbs on its own is not miracle weight-loss strategy, but when combined with the other strategies, can dramatically improve the process.

The Right Timing

If I were to tell you that you could lose weight faster by eating more times throughout the day with little or no exercise, what would you think? Not possible, right? The concept of eating more times throughout the day to lose weight is not new. In fact, it is more natural for us to eat this way than it is to follow the three-square meals per day paradigm most of us were taught to follow as children.

You might find the concept difficult to grasp hold of, but eating four, five, six times, or more times during the day can help you stabilize and maintain a healthier weight – but not the way you might think. We've been conditioned our entire lives to believe less is better when it comes to losing and maintaining weight, and as a result of this conditioning, many of us are under the misconception that eating more than three times per day will negatively impact our weight-loss and stabilization efforts. But this couldn't be further from the truth if you're eating right.

In fact, eating three square meals per day is one of many reasons we gain weight. Going for long periods between meals leads us to overeating and craving foods known to add on the pounds. Not to mention, there is little evidence to suggest that this practice is the best or healthiest way for us to eat.

On the other hand, consuming meals and snacks in timed intervals has a number of positive effects on weight management. It helps to improve sustainability by staving off cravings and hunger, and it supplies a steady stream of nutrients and energy for the body use throughout the day. It decreases the potential for overindulging during meals, and it can minimize the effects of ghrelin, the hunger hormone.

Another positive is that it takes energy to digest the foods we consume. The body produces heat when digesting certain foods like fats, proteins, and complex carbs, which require more time to digest; and the longer your body works, the more calories you burn in the process. Some might argue that the energy expended in negligible, but remember that it's not the one who wins the war, it's the many. And when the foods we consume are carefully selected, not only can they help to support a healthy gut biome but they can also increase the calories expended during the digestive process.

How it all works is this: as your stomach begins to empty, it starts to shrink – similar to when you let the air out of a balloon – which triggers the secretion of ghrelin, the hunger hormone, by specialized cells in the fundus, or upper part of the stomach. As explained in Part I, one of ghrelin's actions is to boost your appetite and stimulate your desire to eat, which normally happens three to four hours after eating. The key to minimizing ghrelin's effects is to control the amount of ghrelin being secreted by the stomach. Unfortunately, there's no on/off switch, so you have to learn to work the system. When you consume regular meals for breakfast, lunch, and dinner, and smaller snacks in between, each separated by a few hours, you are refilling the stomach just as it begins to empty, which stretches the lining of the stomach and limits the secretion of ghrelin.

Now, you must understand this: As much as eating multiple times throughout the day can help you lose and stabilize a healthier weight, it is equally effective in causing weight gain if you're not careful about what you are eating. Overindulging, eating the wrong foods, in the wrong combinations, and at the wrong time of day will help you pack on the pounds, which is why it's so important to understand how your body responds to the foods you eat.

For instance, many of us snack before bedtime. But did you know that if you consume carbs, starches, and sugary snacks at night, you're helping the body store fat? But if you consume a protein snack before going to bed your body will burn calories because it has to work harder through the night to digest the protein?

Spacing your meals and snacks approximately three hours apart usually does the trick, and it's easy enough to employ because you already have a scheduled time of day when you normally eat breakfast, lunch, and dinner. You may have to juggle your schedule a little, but other than that, all you have to do is minimize the mixing and work in a few healthy snacks that support sustainability and optimal digestion. That way, you are well on the road to optimizing your ability to process and assimilate the foods you consume into fat-burning energy.

Now, just to be clear, when I first applied this strategy to my weight-loss efforts, I employed the strategies shared in this chapter. I did not mix simple carbs and animal proteins during meals. I limited sugar intake to iced coffee with hazelnut and vanilla creamer, and to chocolate or peanut butter and oats fiber bars, with the occasional piece of chocolate. As I was in weight-loss mode, I also limited my consumption of carbs and I consumed only healthy whole foods like chicken, lean grass-fed beef, turkey, fish, shellfish, and pork, plus fiber-rich veggies and salad for lunch and dinner – but not just any salad.

Salads are great to experiment with. You can add just about anything to satisfy your palate. Any combination of nuts, seeds, fruits, berries, melons, meats, and cheese with mixed greens can turn the bland into Bam! The portion size for meat, poultry, and fish was anywhere between a quarter and half a pound per serving, and there was no limit to the quantity of veggies and salad consumed.

When I was in the mood for carbs, like pasta, rice, potatoes, or bread, I consumed them as part of a separate meal spaced no less than 2 ½ hours from the time of my last meal or snack. This works especially well in weight-loss mode, which is when you want to avoid mixing proteins and carbs.

Now, because I am an early riser, I often had two breakfasts or included an extra snack, which meant it was not uncommon for me to eat seven times during the day. That sounds like a lot, I know, but it was eating this way that helped me shed 40 pounds twice as fast as I could have done using any traditional weight-loss strategy – and with zero exercise to boot!

Adding healthy snacks between meals offers the perfect opportunity to support a healthy gut biome and satisfy your craving for sweet, salty, and crunchy at the same time. Eating one, or any combination, of protein and fiber-rich nuts and seeds, polyphenol-rich fruits and berries, probiotic yogurts or kefir, apples or bananas with almond or peanut butter, and/or a fiber bar will help satisfy your cravings for sweet, salty, and or crunchy, will keep you satiated, and will work to promote normal energy levels.

A word of caution, though, about fiber bars: Fiber bars are a great way to satisfy your cravings for something sweet, however many fiber bars advertised as healthy snacks (because they contain oats and fiber) are loaded with sugar, which will negatively influence your weight and waistline. Be sure to check the nutritional facts/information panel. Fiber bars should have 20% or more of the daily recommended allowance of fiber, and the percentage of carbs and sugars should not exceed the daily percentage of fiber. Otherwise, it's no better than eating candy with a little fiber in it.

The bottom line is this: when done right, eating a combination of healthy meals and snacks throughout the day can help to:

- Support efficient digestion and a healthy gut biome.
- Promote normal energy levels.
- Minimize hunger and keep you satiated.
- Improve sustainability.
- Satisfy your cravings.
- Help to accelerate and improve your results.

Poly ... What?

You've seen the word *polyphenols* used throughout this book, so what are they? Polyphenols are among the most powerful allies to your weight-loss and management efforts. They are natures antioxidants, powerful micronutrients we get from plant based food sources. They are part of a group of phytochemicals that occur naturally in plants, which provide the abundance of rich colors to the spices, veggies, fruits, and berries we eat and act to protect the produce we consume from damaging UV light and other airborne toxins.

The antioxidant properties of polyphenols also protect our cells from being damaged by increasing numbers of free radicals, but their service to our bodies doesn't stop there. Polyphenols work to prevent the foods we eat from turning into fat, increase the metabolism, and help with the conversion of unhealthy white, or visceral fat, into healthy brown fat we use for energy. They also have a prebiotic action that works to support healthy gut bacteria, and they have powerful anti-inflammatory qualities.

There are three main types of phytochemicals; carotenoids associated with vitamin A, allyl sulfides which are found in garlic and onions, and polyphenols, which are the most abundant of the three with over 500 hundred different types.[20] Those types are broken down further into:

- Phenolic acids, which are found in tea, coffee, blueberries, kiwis, plums, apples, and cherries.
- Flavonoids, which work as both antioxidants and anti-inflammatory agents.
- Stilbenes, which are made mostly of resveratrol, which is the most common, and is found in red wine, red grapes, and peanuts.

- Lignins, which we get from flaxseeds, pumpkin seeds, cranberries, tea, and whole grains, and in varying degrees from cereals, grains, fruits, algae (spirulina), legumes, and some vegetables.

Of course, being a weight-loss superpower, a tremendous amount of research has been done on the health benefits they provide. In weight loss and maintenance, few things come close to the benefits polyphenol-rich foods provide the body. Adding polyphenol-rich foods to your dietary intake will help the following:

- Block the formation of new fat cells.

- Help break down and convert the bad white fat clinging to your belly, hips, neck, and thighs into healthy brown fat we use for energy.

- Support a healthy balance of positive and negative bacteria in the gut.

- Decrease systemic inflammation, (minimize bloating) caused by ingesting carbs, sugars, and salt.

- Protect the body against free radicals, or the toxic by-products of oxygen metabolism, which can cause severe damage to cells and is responsible for causing a multitude of illnesses, as well as promoting aging.

Blueberries are among the most body-benefiting polyphenol-rich foods on the planet, which is likely why they are referenced in so many studies. In fact, many nutritionists feel that if you were going to change one thing about your diet, adding blueberries would be the thing to do.

But if blueberries don't float your boat, there are plenty of places to get your fill of polyphenols. Red grapes and green tea are weight-management rock stars. Both are loaded with polyphenols. And if these are not your cup of tea, either, here is a list of polyphenol-rich foods you can add to your dietary intake. Adding one or two will help, but if you're looking to shed those unwanted pounds and inches, and hold onto your results, more is better.

Veggies

- Artichokes
- Asparagus
- Endive
- Olives (red and green)
- Onions (red and yellow)
- Potatoes (avoid mixing with animal proteins)
- Red leaf lettuce
- Shallots

- Spinach
- Broccoli
- Beets (hi carbs and sugar)

- Spirulina
- Broccoli rabe

Fruits

- Blueberries
- Raspberries
- Cherries (sweet and tart)
- Apples
- Nectarines
- Red grapes
- Pears
- Peaches
- Black elderberries

- Blackberries
- Strawberries
- Plums
- Black currants
- Concord grapes
- Carrots
- Apricots
- Oranges
- Pomegranate

Juices (No Sugar Added)

- Orange juice
- Grapefruit juice
- Pomegranate juice

- Apple juice
- Lemon juice*

_____

*Lemon juice can be added to water as a prebiotic, added to beverages for flavoring, used in juicing recipes, and tastes great in salad dressings.

Legumes, Nuts, and Seeds

- Black beans
- White beans
- Hazelnuts (filberts)
- Walnuts
- Pistachios
- Pumpkin seeds
- Roasted soya nuts

- Red beans
- Lentils
- Almonds
- Pecans
- Chestnuts
- Sunflower seeds
- Flaxseed

On the Spicy Side

- Ginger
- Cinnamon
- Curry powder
- Oregano (dried)
- Rosemary (dried)
- Peppermint (dried)
- Cocoa powder
- Celery seed
- Lemon verbena
- Cumin
- Star anise
- Capers
- Saffron
- Thyme (dried)
- Spearmint (dried)
- Capers
- Sage (dried)

Fats

- Extra-virgin olive oil
- Sesame oil
- Dark chocolate

The Things That Make Our Day

- Coffee
- Tea
- Green tea

And Our Nights

- Red wine
  - Pinot Noir
  - Merlot
  - Cabernet Sauvignon
  - Malbec

As you can see, there are an abundance of polyphenol-rich foods, beverages, and spices you can choose from. Try them all in your favorite recipes.

Bulking Up to Trim Down

Mention fiber supplementation to some people, and they'll look at you like you've got three heads: "I don't need fiber – My grandparents take it." And maybe they do, but it's important to remember that with age comes wisdom. And you don't want to miss out on a powerful weight-management ally.

Fiber isn't just for grandma and grandpa anymore!

It would be foolish to believe that fiber supplementation is anything but what it is: a way to augment dietary fiber intake that promotes healthy digestion, a healthy gut biome, and the elimination of potentially harmful toxins, pathogens, and the unusable by-products of digestion.

Dietary fiber is the fiber we get from the foods we consume. Unfortunately, the standard diet has changed dramatically over the years, and fiber supplementation has become increasingly important for people of all ages. Hectic lifestyles find us consuming increasing amounts of empty-calorie fast-foods, take-outs, and convenience foods with limited nutritional value and fiber content. And while grabbing something on the go may be necessary at times to keep up with a fast-paced life, the grab-on-the-go food options are typically less healthy, provide limited amounts of dietary fiber, and do little to help sustain a healthier weight and waistline.

Today, the average person gets less than half the recommended amount of dietary fiber from the foods consumed – just 14 to 15 grams of fiber per day, when the recommended daily values for women under the age of fifty call for 25 grams per day; for men, it's 30 to 38 grams per day,[21] depending on caloric intake. These values decrease for women and men over the age of fifty to 21 grams for women, and 28- 30 grams for men.[22] Nutritional research, and countless studies have shown the benefits of consuming a diet high in fiber, but getting enough dietary fiber from our foods is proving to be a difficult task, making supplementing your fiber intake a healthy choice.

There are two basic types of fiber – soluble and insoluble – each of which plays an important role in maintaining the health of your digestive system and contributes to your weight-loss and maintenance efforts. *Insoluble fiber* has a more mechanical function in digestion. It does not dissolve when mixed with gastric juices, nor is it affected by the body's natural bacterial flora. Instead, it adds the bulk needed to help keep the intestine clean, and healthy, and helps to regulate bowel movements.

Also called "roughage," insoluble fiber acts like a sponge to absorb water. As it does, it expands inside your stomach, helping you to feel satiated, which helps to delay the secretion of the hunger hormone, ghrelin. Then, as insoluble fiber moves through the digestive system, it helps to remove waste, toxins, undigested and indigestible foods, and other by-products of digestion the body has no use for, which are then expelled from the body when you evacuate your bowels.

Soluble fiber, on the other hand, works a little differently. It mixes with fluids and digestive enzymes in the stomach and forms a gel that can help limit the assimilation of unhealthy substances passing through the intestine. It acts as a prebiotic, and contributes to supporting a healthy balance of positive and negative bacteria in the gut, as well as slows the emptying of your stomach, which also keeps you feeling fuller for longer.

Together, soluble, and insoluble fiber are an asset to your weight-loss and stabilization efforts, and they work to regulate bowel function, reduce cholesterol and triglycerides, aid in managing blood sugar, and strengthen the walls of the intestine, not to mention the cardiovascular benefits they also provide.

If your intent to lose pounds and maintain a healthier weight is for health and longevity reasons, increasing your dietary fiber intake can go a long way. In a Harvard study of over 40,000 male health professionals, researchers found that a high dietary fiber intake was linked to a 40% lower risk of coronary heart disease, versus those with low-fiber intake.[23] Research also strongly suggests that fiber helps to prevent insulin resistance – a condition common to pre-diabetics, and the overweight and obese.

Supplemental Fiber

There is no shortage of fiber supplements in the marketplace; however, all are not equal. To make fiber supplements more palatable and appealing, many manufacturers add food coloring, fructose, or artificial sweeteners like aspartame, which can offset the benefits of fiber to a degree.

Electing to use a fiber supplement is an excellent way to support your weight-management efforts, but it is advisable to go with more natural fiber supplements. Products like natural psyllium husk made from the plantago ovata seed can be difficult for first-timers to handle, however. You might wish to consider starting with a commercial brand, and then mix in increasing amounts of pure psyllium husk over time until you find the balance of fiber and flavor that suits your palate. This will help you accommodate to the flavor and effects of pure fiber, and will minimize the intake of sweeteners. You can also opt for all-natural flavored fiber supplements available at health food stores.

Manufacturers commonly recommend taking fiber three times per day; however, you don't want to overdo it, especially if you are adding fiber-rich foods to your dietary intake at the same time. Too much fiber can result in dry compacted stool, which can be difficult and painful to pass. Starting slow with one or two half-doses per day over the course of a few days will help your body adjust to the increase in fiber intake and will minimize the potential for undesirable side effects.

Note: before you begin to supplement your fiber intake, be sure to read the instructions carefully! Taking a fiber supplements may interfere with the proper assimilation of medications. Most fiber products recommend a window of two hours between the consumption of medicines and that of fiber. Consult with your physician if you are taking prescribed medications for any reason before adding fiber supplements to your diet, and always remember to read the instructions carefully on any fiber supplement you take.

It's important to understand that fiber supplements do not counteract all of the negative effects of poor dietary choices. It doesn't work that way. If it did, we could all eat what we want, when we want, and as much as we want, without consequence – just by taking fiber. Fiber taken before meals may help to decrease caloric intake by limiting the amount of food you consume, but it is not the cure-all for poor eating habits.

Dietary Fiber

Natural sources of fiber are derived from parts of the cell walls of certain grains, fruits, and vegetables, as well as from nuts and seeds, cereals, beans, and other legumes. Listed here are a few of the many fiber-rich foods, including the percentage of daily value per serving which, when added to your diet, can help improve the results of your weight-management efforts.

Fiber Rich Fruit	% Daily Value	Fiber Rich Fruit	% Daily Value
Passion fruit	25g/cup 98% DV	Avocado	13g/avocado 54% DV
Guava	9g/cup 36% DV	Raspberries	8g/cup 32 % DV
Blackberries	8g/cup 31% DV	Pomegranate	7g/cup 28% DV
Persimmon	6g/each 24% DV	Kiwi	5g/cup 22% DV
Pears	4g/cup 17% DV	Oranges	4g/cup 17% DV
Blueberries	4g/cup 14% DV	Tangerines	4g/cup 14% DV
Strawberries	3g/cup 13% DV	Cherries	3g/cup 13% DV
Apricots	3g/cup 12% DV	Bananas	3g/cup 12% DV
Starfruit	3g/cup 12% DV	Apples	3g/cup 12% DV
Mango	3g/cup 11% DV	Grapefruit	3g/cup 10% DV

Fiber Rich Veggies	% Daily Value	Fiber Rich Veggies	% Daily Value
Lima beans	9g/C cooked 37% DV	Acorn squash	9g/C cooked 36% DV
Green peas	9g/C cooked 35% DV	Collard greens	8g/C cooked 30% DV
Artichokes	7g/Medium 28% DV	Butternut squash	7g/C cooked 26% DV
Parsnip	7g/C 26% DV	Broccoli	5g/C cooked 21% DV
Carrots	5g/C cooked 19% DV	Spinach	4g/C cooked 17% DV
Beet greens	4g/C cooked 17% DV	Brussels sprouts	4g/C cooked 16% DV
Green beans	4g/C cooked 16% DV	Okra	4g/C cooked 16% DV
Sweet potatoes	4g/C cooked 16% DV	Swiss chard	4g/C cooked 15% DV
White potato	4g/Medium 15% DV	Asparagus	4g/C cooked 14% DV
Button mushrooms	3g/C cooked 14% DV	Turnips	3g/C cooked 12% DV
Rutabagas	3g/C cooked 12% DV	Corn	3g/C 12% DV
Fennel	3g/C 11% DV	Kale	3g/C cooked 10% DV

Other fruits, and veggies containing less than 2g of fiber per serving include watermelon, cantaloupe, pineapple, grapes, plums, papaya, lychees, peaches and nectarines, tomatoes, zucchini, eggplant, cabbage, bell peppers, cauliflower, celery, leeks, and lettuce.[24]

Excellent sources of fiber include:

- White beans
- Navy beans
- Lima beans
- Black beans
- Red beans
- Pinto beans
- Chickpeas
- Lentils
- Peas (sweet)
- Walnuts
- Pecans
- Almonds
- Pistachios
- Air-popped popcorn

- High-fiber cereals
- Edamame
- Brown rice
- Wild rice
- Barley
- Sunflower seeds
- Pumpkin seeds
- Flax seeds
- Chia seeds
- Whole-grain breads
- Seven-grain breads
- Pumpernickel
- Cracked wheat
- Dark rye bread

The Skinny on Juicing

Juicing is a favorite among many dieters. It's a flavorful way to get the antioxidant benefits of polyphenol-rich foods in liquid form. Juicing began to grow in popularity in the 1970s with the health and fitness craze, but it wasn't until recently that we could derive all the benefits of juicing.

In the 70s, most juicers extracted the juice from fruits and veggies by fracturing the cell walls, and separated out the fiber-rich pulp, and skin, which led to some controversy over the benefits of juicing. Opponents contended that stripping healthy whole foods of fiber was not to our benefit, and supporters pushed the enzyme, vitamin and mineral agenda. Few if any mentioned the sugar content.

Today, juicing is a different game, and it's a welcome ally to weight management. High-speed blenders liquefy whole foods – skin, pulp, and all – which provides the vitamins, minerals, and antioxidant benefits of the polyphenol-rich whole foods we are juicing, as well as maintaining the benefits of some of the fiber.

Additionally, juicing can be used for detox diets, a between meal boost, or just a healthier way to refresh yourself. Plus, adding flavors like maca powder and cocoa boost the nutritional content and fiber value while improving taste.

Other Beneficial Beverages

There's no denying that we love our caffeine. Everyday around the world over 2.25 billion cups of coffee, and twice that amount of tea is poured and enjoyed. In the United States alone, we start our days with over 400 million cups of joe[25] and consume 1.42 million pounds of tea (mostly iced). Beginning the day just wouldn't be the same without our coffee or tea. They are the world's get-up-and-go beverages. Despite coffee having over two times the caffeine of tea, both offer a morning pick-me-up that helps kick us into gear.

But waking us up is not all our favorite caffeinated beverages do for us. They also help to temporarily boost the metabolism, which lets us burn a few more calories. But don't go betting the farm on the long-term weight-loss benefits of caffeine. Although caffeine does help boost the metabolism, its effects are temporary, and studies suggest the body can build a tolerance to it in as little as one to two weeks.[26] Even with very high doses, its ability to increase alertness will diminish within eighteen days, and when it does, its metabolism-boosting effects diminish with it.[27]

It is possible to reduce your tolerance to caffeine if so afflicted, but doing so is much like cyclical dieting. You might have better luck swimming up Niagara Falls than getting passionate coffee and tea drinkers to give up their morning brew for two weeks just to decrease their tolerance to caffeine. However, this doesn't mean your weight-management efforts can't benefit from your favorite caffeinated beverages.

Tea and coffee benefit your weight-management efforts in other ways. Both are high in fat-blocking polyphenols, and will help to prevent fat storage, as well as assist in converting unsightly white fat into healthy brown fat we use for energy. So, drink up and enjoy, and if you want a little more bang from your caffeine buck, try mixing things up a bit.

Try a different brand of coffee. Coffee beans grown at higher altitudes are generally higher in fat-burning polyphenols. Or during the day, throw in a few cups of green tea, with honey and/or lemon (hot or iced). This way you get the best of both worlds. You can enjoy your morning brew, and you benefit from the fat-burning power of green tea as well.

Green tea gets its well-deserved reputation as a fat burner because it has a combination of caffeine and an abundance of powerful fat-burning flavonoids (polyphenols), which together can reduce body fat (especially stubborn belly fat) by up to 19%.[28]

One cup of green tea has just two (2) calories – or 23 calories with a teaspoon of honey and a squeeze of lemon – provides the prebiotic actions of lemon juice, a mild metabolic boost from the caffeine, and the fat-burning power of four powerful catechins: epigallocatechin gallate (EGCG), epigallocatechin (EGC), epicatechin gallate (ECG), and epicatechin (EC),[29] making green tea the perfect complement to your weight-loss and stabilization efforts.

If green tea isn't your thing, steeping a cup of traditional black tea, the most commonly consumed tea on the planet, will help your efforts as well. Black, white, oolong, and green teas are all harvested from the same shrub, *Camellia sinensis*, and are equally endowed with a generous portion of polyphenols. The only difference is that black teas have been oxidized more.

Choices in Alcohol

The fact is, alcohol consumption can cause weight gain, especially if you eat while drinking. It slows the motility of the digestive tract, and can lead to a decrease in the secretion of digestants.[30] Alcohol not only stimulates the appetite but it also changes how the body metabolizes and stores the calories you consume, causing them to be stored as fat. And if the alcohol being consumed is sugar, carb, and or calorie-rich, like beer, sweet wines, and flavored liquors, you are promoting weight gain, and contributing to your weight management struggles.

Alcohol can slow your weight-loss efforts, and if weight loss is your goal, you might want to hold off or minimize consumption until you reach your target weight. This is aside from the fact that alcohol breaks down into a highly toxic compound called acetaldehyde, a known carcinogen.[31] This carcinogen can contribute to a number of health issues. Alcohol also interferes with the body's ability to process and assimilate the foods we consume, not to mention that overconsumption can lead to unwise dietary choices.

However, life doesn't stop just because you're on a diet, and if you are going to enjoy the occasional libation, remember a few simple things that can help minimize the damage. First, dry red wines can actually benefit your weight-loss efforts. Each 5-ounce serving will set you back about 125 calories. But red wines, which are typically low in sugar, have an abundance of polyphenols that can help offset systemic inflammation and the dietary bloat associated with the consumption of carb-rich foods.

Red wines made with grapes harvested from higher altitudes tend to have a higher concentration of polyphenols, despite the loss of some during the fermentation process. Among the best for weight management are Pinot Noir, Cabernet Sauvignon, Merlot, and Malbec. All are dry, and all offer a variety of rich full flavors. The "Rule of Red" in weight loss is to avoid sweet wines, sangrias, and flavored wines.

What about hard liquor? All alcohol has calories, plain and simple, so when you consume it, your body must first burn the calories from the alcohol before it can get back to burning the calories from the foods you've consumed. So, the rules for alcohol consumption are simple. Hard liquor should be consumed straight, or mixed with water and/or plain soda water. Adding sugary mixes will spike the sugar levels and negatively influence any weight-loss efforts, and although some suggest artificially sweetened diet beverages can be mixed with your favorites, consider the effects artificial sweeteners have on the body. Lowering inhibitions, and stimulating cravings at the same time in not a winning combination.

Your safest bet while losing weight and maintaining your weight is to avoid sugar-rich flavored alcohols. Stick with the basics straight scotch, bourbon, whisky, vodka, gin, or rum, as they have no significant carb or sugar content, with one exception. Studies have identified a type of natural sugar called agavin, which comes from the agave plant and is used to make tequila. It can actually lower blood glucose levels and help us lose weight. Different from the sweetener known as agave syrup, agavins are indigestible and do not raise blood sugar levels.[32]

What about beer? There's nothing like a cold beer on a hot day, at a ballgame, a picnic, the beach, or barbeque, but the bottom line is that beer is not your friend when you're trying to lose weight. Carbs, alcohol, and lowered inhibitions are a triple threat to your weight-management efforts. If you must – enjoy them sensibly, and understand the negative influence it will have on your weight loss efforts.

Chapter Summary

- Pre- and Probiotics are essential to supporting a healthy gut biome.

- Separating or minimizing the mixing of animal proteins and simple carbohydrates at mealtime will help improve the efficiency by which you process and assimilate the foods you consume.

- Eating more often throughout the day can help you lose, stabilize, and maintain a healthier weight and waistline.

- Polyphenol-rich foods are powerful allies in your weight-management efforts.

- Fiber supplementation improves digestive health and efficiency, and is necessary to augment dietary fiber intake in accord with today's changing dietary habits.

- Beneficial beverages add flavor to your life and support your weight-management efforts.

10

The Food in You

Nutritional science has come a long way since 1848, when German physician Julius Mayer suggested that food was the body's source of energy, and that our ability to function was not something solely of divine origin. I can only imagine the controversy this notion created in the scientific and religious communities of the time. But despite what is likely to have been strong opposition from those unwilling to accept his suggestion, his premise changed the way the world looks the food we consume.

Since then, every food we consume has been broken down into its smallest components to determine how it affects the body when ingested, and this information, in part, has been used to develop the weight-loss and dieting strategies used by consumers around the world.

The science is sound; however, the weight-loss and dieting strategies often fail to look at the bigger picture and use only bits and pieces of this information in developing their singularly focused strategies to help us lose weight, which is much like teaching someone to bake a cake with flour and water, and forgetting to mention the butter, milk, sugar, salt, baking powder, and vanilla also needed to get the job done.

Food Basics

Whether attempting to lose unwanted pounds and inches, or maintain your weight, it's not enough to simply say that fat is bad for you or carbs are the reason you gain weight, and then eliminate them from your diet. This approach has proven to do more harm than good. Having a basic understanding of how the foods you consume affect the body, and how they can either help or interfere with your ability to manage a healthier weight and waistline is the major theme of this book. So, at this point, let's review a few basic facts about food and nutrition.

The body requires three types of food or macronutrients to function efficiently: protein, fat, and carbohydrates. The percentage of dietary intake of each varies depending on which site you reference; however, generally accepted daily guidelines established by the Food and Nutrition Board, a subgroup of the Institute of Medicine, are as follows: protein, 10 – 35%, fat, 10 – 35%, and carbohydrates, 45 – 65%.

Proteins

The body benefits in a number of ways from the consumption of proteins. They are necessary to our existence because they provide the body with amino acids, the body's building blocks used to grow, repair, or replace the cells and tissues in the body, and they contribute to the production of enzymes, hormones, and other chemicals the body requires to function efficiently.

Proteins are more complex than other foods, and require a lot of energy to digest. Upwards of 30% of the calories derived from the consumption of protein is burned during the digestion process.[33] Proteins are also satiating, which is to say they keep you feeling fuller longer.

It takes between three and six hours for your stomach to empty after consumption, which is helpful in keeping the stomach stretched and the secretion of ghrelin, the hunger hormone, down to a minimum, adding benefit to your weight-management efforts. Good sources of protein can be found in;

- Grass-fed beef*
- Lamb*
- Poultry (skin off)

- Lentils
- Chickpeas
- Beans – black, white, red, kidney

- Fish
- Pork*
- Eggs*
- Cheese*
- Dairy*

- Spirulina
- Quinoa
- Nuts and seeds
- Nut Butters – almond and peanut
- Certain sprouted grains

*When choosing animal-based (protein) products for consumption, it is important to consider the fat content and portion size. Choosing lean cuts of meat, skinless chicken, turkey, and lean cuts of pork will best serve your weight-management needs and help minimize intake of unhealthy fats.

Fats

Before carbs were the focus of the health, fitness, and weight-loss industries, it was fat. Unfortunately, the well-intended, but misguided use of clinical research data left fat with a bad rep that has carried over for many years, despite the importance of dietary fat for the body.

A common misconception among dieters is that all dietary fat is bad. As a result, dieters often attempt to restrict or eliminate all fat when dieting, which can prove to be a costly mistake for your weight-loss and management efforts. Fat stores and supplies the body with a usable energy source. It helps in the absorption certain nutrients, and it supports cell growth, as well as providing warmth and insulation to protect vital organs. It also plays an important role in the production of certain hormones, some of which are key to regulating appetite and others which help metabolize fat.

When it comes to fat, just like anything else there's both good and bad. Bad fats are the saturated and trans fats that are being consumed in increasing amounts today. They contribute to weight gain, raise your LDL (bad cholesterol), and contribute to cardiovascular disease. Saturated fats can be found in abundance in grain-fed and fatty cuts of beef, dark-meat poultry, poultry skin, pork, whole milk, cheese, butter, processed foods, deli meats, sausages, bacon, hot dogs, fast foods, and the like.

Trans fats are those you see listed on product nutrition labels as "Partially Hydrogenated Oils." They result from a food processing method called hydrogenation. Trans fats were added to foods to enhance flavor, texture, and shelf life; however, since the push to ban unhealthy trans fats from foods was initiated, companies have been removing added trans fats from their products, but this doesn't mean we are free and clear of them. We also get them from the following:[34]

- fried foods (french fries, doughnuts, deep-fried fast foods)
- margarine (stick and tub)
- vegetable shortening
- baked goods (cookies, cakes, pastries)
- processed snack foods (crackers, microwave popcorn)
- breakfast sandwiches and biscuits

The latest dietary guidelines recommended by the Mayo Clinic is to keep consumption of saturated fats below 10% of dietary intake, and consumption of trans fats at less than 1%. It's not likely you will be able to eliminate them completely, but keeping them, below recommended levels is in your best interest, both health and weight wise.

The good fats, or unsaturated fats, are polyunsaturated and mono-unsaturated fats that contain omega 3 and omega 6 fatty acids. These are important because although the body can synthesize most fats from the diet, it can't synthesize omega 3 and omega 6,[35] which means you must get them from the foods you consume.

Omega 3 fatty acids are helpful in preventing inflammation and heart disease. Combined with other omega fatty acids, they can reduce triglycerides (fat in the blood stream), prevent arterial plague formation, and help manage blood pressure. They also support healthy skin and provide the skins with its natural oil barrier, which helps to keep skin hydrated, plumper, and younger looking. Omega 3s and omega 6s can be found in lean cuts of grass-fed beef, skin-off poultry, fish, fish oil, nuts, seeds, canola, olive oils, and avocados.

Note: Omega fatty acids are essential to the body, but before dosing yourself with supplemental omega fatty acids, understand that the body requires a specific ratio of omegas. Too much of either one can result in certain health issues. It is always advisable to discuss supplementation with your nutritionist prior to starting.

Most fat in your diet comes in the form of triglycerides. Once assimilated, the triglycerides are broken down and stored as free fatty acids in your liver, or as body fat, or are used by muscle tissue as a source of energy during physical activity. The key for weight management is to maintain your daily intake of fats to the middle to lower end of the recommended 10 –35% of healthy fats, and to minimize your consumption of unhealthy trans fats (hydrogenated oils) and saturated fats. By maintaining your intake of healthy fats at these levels, you support healthy blood triglyceride (blood fat) levels, which helps prevent leptin resistance, or a decrease in sensitivity to leptin.

Carbohydrates

Like fats, carbs have gotten a bad rep over the years. When everyone realized eliminating fat from the diet was responsible for a dramatic increase in overweight and obesity across the nation, it was easy to point the weight gain finger of blame instead at carbohydrates.

Carbs are the body's main source of energy, and they contain "hidden sugars" that are used to fuel your brain, organs, and nervous system. In order to fulfill the body's energy demands, the recommended dietary intake of carbs is between 45 and 65%, or nearly two-thirds of your daily caloric intake.

Carbs are made up of three components: sugar, starch (both sugars), and fiber. When consumed, they break down into smaller sugars like glucose, fructose, and sucrose, which are readily absorbed and used as energy. What isn't used for energy is first converted to glycogen and is stored in the liver, and muscle tissue. When the liver and muscle tissue have reached their capacity to store glycogen, which on average is about 400 grams for muscle tissue and 100 grams for the liver, or the equivalent of just over 1-pound worth, the remaining glucose in glycogen is stored as fat.

There are two types of carbs most dieters are familiar with: simple and complex. Both are sugars, but each responds very differently in the body when consumed. Simple carbs are digested, converted to basic sugar or glucose, and are absorbed rapidly. Because they are quickly assimilated, consuming simple carbs causes blood sugar levels to spike within 45 minutes, and then remain elevated for approximately two hours. This leads to fluctuations in energy levels and promotes weight gain if the energy goes unused.

Simple carbs are sugars that support the proliferation of bad (negative) gut bacteria and cause the body to retain salt and water, which is why we often feel bloated after carb-heavy meals. They are found in foods like:

- Refined potato, wheat, and rice flour (removes the nutrients and fiber)
- Pasta, rice, and potatoes
- Corn syrup
- High fructose corn syrup
- Concentrated fruit juices
- Breads, cakes, cookies, pastries made with refined flour
- Flour-based sugar-free cakes and cookies
- Fruits
- Milk and milk products.
- Candy
- Soft drinks and flavored juices
- Refined sugar
- Raw sugar
- Products containing sugar, corn syrup, high fructose corn syrup, or basically everything we eat from a package

Complex carbs are clusters of sugar molecules bound together with fiber, which slows the digestion process, providing a steady flow or release of glucose, or useable energy, without spiking blood sugar levels. The slow release of sugars helps to benefit to your weight-management efforts. Complex carbs are found in foods like:

- Whole wheat and multigrain breads and cereals
- Barley
- Quinoa
- Yams
- Beans, lentils, peas, chickpeas
- Split peas, kidney, soy, and pinto beans
- Pumpkin
- Nuts and seeds
- Low- fat milk
- Yogurt
- Steel-cut oats and old-fashioned rolled oats
- Long-grain, wild, and basmati rice
- Vegetables (most)
- Squash, zucchini
- Beets
- Whole-grain pastas
- Buckwheat
- Corn
- Soy milk

Simple carbs have been taking the heat for the better part of twenty years or more, but all carbs are not the enemy – not even the bad ones – despite their association with overweight and obesity. If consumed sensibly, they pose little problem to your weight and waistline. The problem is, and always has been, our overconsumption of them. The average person consumes far in excess of the recommended 225 – 325 grams of carbs every day without realizing it.

The foods we consume on a daily basis are loaded with carbs, and hidden sugars. Many of them are foods we have become accustomed to consuming, and we don't think twice about before eating or drinking them. "Carbohydrate" is code for sugar. Sugar is storable energy, and where the body may eliminate an overabundance of other nutrients, it will store as much energy as it can in your fat cells.

A few extra carbs now and then would normally pose little or no threat for those living an active, healthy lifestyle, but when you consider the physical changes occurring in the body that interfere with your ability to process and assimilate the foods you consume, coupled with our hectic lifestyles, poor eating habits, the effects of stress and cortisol, and limited physical activity, you have the major players contributing to your weight-loss and management struggles.

Which brings us back to questioning our eating behaviors. Question your daily intake of bread, sweets, starch based veggies, and sugar- and carb-rich beverages, and see how much fuel you are adding to your weight-loss and management struggles. You might just be surprised how modifying your intake along with optimization techniques will improve your efforts.

For example, the recommended daily intake for sugar is no more than 6 teaspoons for women and 9 teaspoons for men, but the average person consumes two to three times this amount, consuming 19.5 teaspoons of sugar daily, or about 66 pounds each year.[36]

Now, it's not likely you are dumping 19 to-20 teaspoons of sugar in your coffee or tea every day. At least I hope not. This number also reflects the amount of added sugars in other foods, and beverages we are consuming on a daily basis. Sugars we rarely consider are as follows:

Beverage/Serving	Sugar in Grams (Average)	Sugar in Teaspoons
Soda (12-ounce) can	39	9.3
Grape juice	36	8.5
Apple juice	24	5.75
Flavored juice drinks	23	5.5

Beverage/Serving	Sugar in Grams (Average)	Sugar in Teaspoons
Sweetened iced tea	22	5.25.
Pineapple juice	18	4.25
Orange juice	7	1.7

We must also consider that carbs are sugars. One 4-ounce roll contains approximately 60 grams of carbohydrate. One 2-ounce slice of bread or toast contains 30 grams, approximately 15 grams per ounce.[37]

Now, eliminating all carbs from your diet is near impossible, and doing so will dramatically affect the sustainability factor of your weight loss and management efforts. Even the most dedicated dieters will eventually cave to their cravings. The key to enjoying your favorite carbs sensibly comes in knowing how to address the effects they have on the body. Knowing your intake limits as regulated by your level of physical activity and your other dietary habits, and optimizing your ability to process and assimilate them efficiently, allows for the sensible enjoyment of your favorite indulgences.

Does this mean you'll be able to eat cake and pastries every day without having to worry about your waistline? Not likely, but you can enjoy many of your favorites on a regular basis without having to worry about your waistline or permanent weight gain, which is where I believe most dieters want to be.

The bottom line is that we are all a little different when it comes to our tolerance for dieting, our levels of activity, and our eating behaviors. The degree to which each of the barriers, blocks, and changes (BBCs) affects the ability to lose unwanted pounds and maintain a healthier weight and waistline also differs. If you were to take two people living on opposite sides of the same town, with both being the same height and weight and each with the same job description, lifestyle, interests, and activity levels, and you put them on the exact same diet, each would have a different experience. One may have more hunger and cravings then the other. One will lose weight faster than the other, and one will lose more weight than the other, despite consuming the exact same foods.

You would think they would both lose the same amount of weight at the same speed, but they don't because dieting alone does not address the BBCs specific to each of us. The first dieter may handle stress better than the second and have lower levels of circulating cortisol, or the second dieter might be taking medications on a daily basis, or have the need to regularly take antibiotics which interfere with the ability to process food efficiently. It could be any combination of BBCs that will influence the outcome.

The one thing we all have in common is the need to fuel our bodies, and we can't do that effectively without being able to process and assimilate the foods we consume. To do so, you must not only restrict, you must also optimize.

Chapter Summary

- Having a basic understanding of the foods you consume is essential for effective weight loss and weight-management success.
- The three essential macronutrients the body requires are protein, fat, and carbohydrates.
- All three macronutrients are essential for your health, as well as your weight-management efforts.
- Proteins are the body's building blocks.
- 30% of protein calories are used to digest proteins.
- Fats help absorb nutrients, support cell growth, and aid in the production of hormones.
- Fats support healthy skin by providing protective emollients.
- Healthy fats are the unsaturated monounsaturated or polyunsaturated fats.
- Unhealthy fats are saturated fats and trans fats.
- Saturated fats and trans fats contribute to cardiovascular disease, high blood pressure, elevated cholesterol, arterial plaque formation, overweight, and obesity.
- Carbohydrates are hidden sugars.
- Sugar is a sweet-tasting dissolvable form of carbohydrate.
- The average person consumes two to three times more sugar than recommended each day.
- Simple carbs convert to sugar (glucose) quickly and can spike blood sugar levels, resulting in fluctuation of energy levels and weight gain.
- Complex carbs release sugar slowly, providing the body with a steady stream of energy, preventing spiking blood sugar, and helping with weight management.
- There are a number of factors unique to the individual that influence a person's ability to lose weight and maintain a healthy weight.
- Optimization, rather than restricted caloric intake alone, is the most efficient way to manage your weight.

11

Putting It All Together

*Some people want it to happen, some wish it would happen,
others make it happen.*

– Michael Jordan

It's only natural for dieters to want the best of all worlds: a trimmer waistline, normal energy levels, a healthy body, and lasting results from our weight-loss and maintenance efforts, as well as the ability to enjoy favorite foods once the diet has come to an end, without having to worry about expanding waistlines or permanent weight gain. But history has shown this to be an unachievable goal for most.

The promise of lasting results is the illusion we buy into, whether it's our first or our twenty-first diet. It doesn't matter if it's a self-governed, do-it-yourself diet or a program diet. The hope and the desire is there. The effort is made, but achieving lasting results continues to elude 99% of dieters.

The weight-loss and health and fitness industries offer the best products, programs, and equipment they can to reduce caloric intake and/or increase energy expenditure. And although a measure for some wishing to lose weight, on their own these solutions are not enough to deal with the complexities of weight gain.

You now know weight gain is not solely the result of overeating. If that were the case, all you would have to do is lose weight once, and then keep your calorie count at or under the recommended daily intake for your age, sex, and level of activity. But this doesn't happen because weight gain is the result of more than just overeating. To close the gap between the results you are getting now and the results you desire, you need to start with three things.

- Address the pitfalls common to weight-loss and dieting strategies.
- Identify your barriers, blocks, and changes.
- Address the barriers, blocks, and changes.

Addressing the Pitfalls

As you may remember, the pitfalls common to dieting are restriction, sustainability, transitioning, and maintenance. Increasing your meal frequency will help minimize the effects a restricted caloric intake. Alternating healthy meals and snacks in timed intervals lessens the secretion of ghrelin-minimizing hunger and cravings. It also helps provide a steady stream of nutrients throughout the day to support normal energy levels, and with the inclusion of satiating proteins, complex carbs, and healthy fats, can help prevent the body's starvation response from being triggered.

Sustainability is key to success in both weight loss and weight maintenance. Increasing the number of healthy meals and snacks you consume will help with the hunger, and cravings that keep you from sustaining your efforts at weight reduction, but you must also work to minimize or eliminate the effects of leptin – the appetite controlling hormone by including healthy fats in both meals and snacks, as well as satisfying your palate by adding healthier versions (when possible) of some of your favorite foods.

Transitioning from your weight-loss and dieting strategies is crucial to stabilizing and maintaining the hard-earned results of your efforts. It is the bridge between your dieting efforts and your final destination: the active, healthy lifestyle you desire and deserve.

Regardless of whether you are employing a program diet or a self-governed/do-it-yourself diet, minimize the post-diet weight gain by addressing the barriers, blocks, and changes influencing and or interfering with your body's ability to process and assimilate the foods you're consuming. After all, you've worked hard to lose those unwanted pounds and inches.

Slowly reintroduce some of your favorite foods or, preferably, healthier versions of them so that your body can accommodate to the increase in calories from fats, carbs, and sugar. And by reintroducing these foods gradually, you are in a better position to see how each will affect your body.

In order to maintain your results, you must address the barriers, blocks, and changes interfering with your weight-loss and stabilization efforts, if you have not already done so. Indeed, maintaining your post-diet weight is much like taking a long voyage. You've set the course for lifelong mainte-nance. If you should go off course, you make minor adjustments to return and then stay the course. You'll soon find yourself anchored securing in a safe harbor, having achieved success and having learned how to maintain it.

Addressing the BBCs

The "4" in *A Cure 4 Dieting* represents the psychological/emotional, genetic, environmental, and physical barriers I encountered fifteen years ago. In learning to address them, I was able to transform my waistline and my life, but I also changed the way I think about weight and dieting, and it will change the way you think about it, too.

Addressing the psychological or emotional barriers starts with questioning your dietary habits: When you eat, how you eat, and what you eat to determine if your eating behaviors are governed by paradigms, traditions, and routines that do not work in your best interests weight wise, or if overeating is the result of chronically elevated cortisol levels from stress, or the result of the proliferation of negative gut bacteria and the chemical messengers they send to the brain to stimulate cravings for starches, carbs, and sugar-heavy foods.

My journey began simply by questioning: Why I was gaining all the weight back? I found that it wasn't only me – the majority of dieters shared the same experience and had the same question. By questioning your personal dietary habits, eating behaviors, and beliefs about dieting you can update outmoded beliefs with current information. That self-examination will serve you well.

Addressing the emotional aspects of the psychological barrier has more to do with the separation anxiety some dieters feel when they have eliminated certain foods. But here, too, you should start by questioning why you feel the way you do about eliminating these foods from your dietary intake. Consider whether it's simply because the comfort they offer or it's habit; might you be actually addicted to them? Nutritional researchers have discovered certain foods have an addictive quality because when consumed they trigger the release of feel good chemicals from the brain. Indeed, a study at the University of Michigan showed that 7 to 10% of participants had full-blown addictions, and 92% showed signs of addictive-like eating behaviors regarding some the food used in the study.[38]

Milder forms of separation anxiety are easily addressed by including healthier versions of your favorites or adding other foods that equally satisfy your palate and cravings for sweet, bitter, sour, and salty. However, an inability to avoid certain foods for any length of time may suggest a higher level of food addiction, requiring professional help.

The genetic barrier can be surmounted by increasing your intake of polyphenol-rich foods and beverages, which can turn your fat-storing switch off and nullify the workings of the fat genes, FTO, IRX3, and IRX5. These are found in abundance in coffee, tea, green tea, red wine, brightly colored berries, and vegetables, and can be consumed whole or juiced.

Many of the environmental barriers are out of our control, and cannot be directly addressed. We can only work to minimize their effects on our bodies. The environmental barriers accelerate physical changes that interfere with your weight-management efforts and degrade the efficiency of the digestive process. Eating whole foods and following the recommendations in Chapter 6 for avoiding contaminated products will go a long way toward breaking down those environmental barriers.

The physical barriers are the cumulative effects of the BBCs on the body's ability to process and assimilate the foods we consume efficiently. So, addressing them is all about supporting healthy digestion to minimize their effects on your weight, waistline, and overall health.

These formerly unknown adversaries disrupt the healthy balance of microorganisms in the stomach, and can lead to a decrease in the quantity and quality of gastric juices and digestive enzymes, resulting in inefficient digestion of the foods we consume. In essence, they accelerate the degradation of the digestive system

Addressing the physical changes includes adding a variety of pre- and probiotics, and a healthy dose of polyphenol-rich foods spaced evenly throughout the day. Foods and beverages supplemented with probiotics like yogurt and kefir are usually enough support for healthy individuals; higher supplemental dosages may be required for individuals taking antibiotics and other medications on a regular basis, or for those who have increased exposure to environmental toxins and antibacterial chemicals, products and cleaners.

Own it, Don't Rent it

My intent in this book is not to dissuade you from using your chosen methods of weight loss and dieting but, rather, to improve the sustainability and effectiveness of the strategies you employ. When I first discovered the truth about weight loss and dieting, I knew I had the same two choices you have today: accept circumstances as they exist and continue to cycle through periods of weight loss and weight gain or accept responsibility for breaking that cycle.

I accepted responsibility for making the change, and what took years of research and trials to find an effective and efficient alternative to dieting alone, you can begin to apply in fifteen minutes. *A Cure 4 Dieting* brings to your attention the complexities of weight gain and shows how to bring your weight-loss efforts to fruition. Whether you are a seasoned dieter or a beginner, you need to question why you might disregard information that can help you put an end to your weight-loss struggles, and support a healthy immune system with little to no more effort than one of the many diets you would employ during your lifetime.

The point is: Dieting on its own is not the healthy choice we believe it to be. It is an ineffective and inefficient way to manage your weight. It is tedious, time-consuming, frustrating, and directly responsible for causing post-diet weight gain. It promotes cyclical dieting, which has a cost far greater than the money you'll spend to lose the same weight repeatedly.

Just as overweight and obesity steal from us those things in life that are most precious – time, health, memories, money, self-esteem, and the ability to enjoy the active healthy lifestyle we desire and deserve – so too does dieting. The average dieter will sacrifice an unconscionable number of years dealing with hunger, cravings, stress, moodiness, expense, and frustration for results that are temporary at best. It's time to change the paradigm!

Earlier I mentioned that I am not a "That's just the way it is" kind of guy. So, the thought of you not implementing a few simple dietary changes and making a few additions to improve your life doesn't bode well with me. I have no interest in joining the growing numbers of weight-loss gurus. My interest here is only to share what I have discovered and provide you with a means to accelerate and improve the results of your efforts and show you how to make them last. To make things a bit easier for you to implement these ideas, you are invited to visit: https://ACure4Dieting.com where you can download at No Cost to you some helpful resources to aid you in your pursuit of the active healthy lifestyle you desire and deserve – Life is too short to diet more than once my friends. Live strong, live well, live long!

Knowing, not following, is the key to your success.

Endnotes

Part I

1. See https://nutritionj.biomedcentral.com/articles/10.1186/1475-2891-10-9.

2. https://nutritionj.biomedcentral.com/articles/10.1186/1475-2891-10-9

3. http://www.fitnessforweightloss.com/diet-and-weight-loss-statistics/

4. http://www.basicknowledge101.com/subjects/brain.html

5. https://www.vocabulary.com/dictionary/subliminal

6. https://www.wordstream.com/blog/ws/2017/10/24/subliminal-advertising

7. https://nutritionj.biomedcentral.com/articles/10.1186/1475-2891-10-9

8. http://abcnews.go.com/Health/100-million-dieters-20-billion-weight-loss-industry/story?id=16297197

9. https://en.wikipedia.org/wiki/George_Cheyne_(physician)

10, https://en.wikipedia.org/wiki/John_Rollo.

11. https://en.wikipedia.org/wiki/William_Banting

12. www.sciencedaily.com/releases/2006/11/061120060301.htm

13. University of Georgia. "Confusion About Calories Is Nothing New, Professor Finds." *ScienceDaily*. ScienceDaily, 20 November 2006. www.sciencedaily.com/releases/2006/11/061120060301.htm

14. https://en.wikipedia.org/wiki/Lulu_Hunt_Peters

15. https://physicalculturestudy.com/2015/04/22/weight-loss-in-1920s-america-the-reducing-craze/

16. http://www.femalefirst.co.uk/health/length-of-the-average-diet-279944.html

17. https://www.webmd.com/diet/obesity/features/plateau-no-more#1

18. https://www.livestrong.com/article/392832-does-not-eating-slow-your-metabolism/

19. https://www.livestrong.com/article/392832-does-not-eating-slow-your-metabolism/

20. http://www.senescence.info/aging_definition.html

21. https://www.animated-teeth.com/tooth_decay/t3_tooth_decay_remineralization.htm

22. http://www.heart.org/idc/groups/ahamah-public/@wcm/@sop/@smd/documents/downloadable/ucm_470704.pdf

23. http://www.heart.org/idc/groups/ahamah-public/@wcm/@sop/@smd/documents/downloadable/ucm_470704.pdf

24. https://www.nbcnews.com/health/health-news/heavy-burden-obesity-may-be-even-deadlier-thought-f6C10930019

25. http://easo.org/education-portal/obesity-facts-figures/

26. https://www.cdc.gov/media/releases/2012/t0507_weight_nation.html

27. https://nutritionj.biomedcentral.com/articles/10.1186/1475-2891-10-9

28. http://www.dictionary.com/browse/middle-age-spread

29. https://www.health24.com/Medical/Flu/Preventing-flu/your-gut-is-the-cornerstone-of-your-immune-system-20160318

30. https://www.webmd.com/diet/obesity/features/the-facts-on-leptin-faq#1

31. http://www.yourhormones.info/hormones/ghrelin/

32. https://www.dosomething.org/us/facts/11-facts-about-american-eating-habits

33. http://sugarscience.ucsf.edu/the-growing-concern-of-overconsumption.html#.W2xcb9JKjIU

34. https://www.healthline.com/nutrition/is-leaky-gut-real#section2

35. https://nutritionreview.org/2018/03/gastric-balance-heartburn-caused-excess-acid/

36. https://www.gdx.net/product/intestinal-permeability-assessment-urine

37. http://www.heart.org/HEARTORG/HealthyLiving/HealthyKids/ChildhoodObesity/Overweight-in-Children_UCM_304054_Article.jsp#.WxlFwUgvzIU

38. http://www.geneticlifehacks.com/weight-loss-genetics-fto-polymorphisms/

39. http://www.basicknowledge101.com/subjects/brain.html

40. https://www.simplypsychology.org/unconscious-mind.html

41. https://www.simplypsychology.org/unconscious-mind.html

42. https://jamesclear.com/new-habit

43. https://www.brainyquote.com/quotes/w_clement_stone_193778

44. https://www.livescience.com/22728-pollution-facts.html

45. https://www.msn.com/en-in/health/wellness/countries-with-the-most-obese-kids/ss-AAjaOig?fullscreen=true#image=2

46. https://www.bbc.com/news/magazine-20243692

47. https://nutritionj.biomedcentral.com/articles/10.1186/1475-2891-10-9

48. http://kidshealth.org/en/parents/breastfeed-often.html

49. https://www.helpguide.org/articles/stress/stress-symptoms-signs-and-causes.htm

50. https://www.prevention.com/weight-loss/g20439118/how-to-prevent-weight-gain-due-to-stress-and-anxiety/

51. http://www.miamiherald.com/living/article1961770.html

52. https://www.activebeat.com/your-health/7-most-common-stress-related-health-problems/7/

53. http://www.todaysdietitian.com/newarchives/111609p38.shtml

54. https://www.telegraph.co.uk/news/science/7881819/Smell-of-jasmine-as-calming-as-valium.html

55. https://www.up-nature.com/blogs/news/top-17-best-essential-oils-for-stress-and-anxiety-and-how-to-use-them

56. https://www.verywellfit.com/health-benefits-of-different-physical-activity-levels-3496010

57. https://newatlas.com/global-antibiotic-use-rising/53963/

58. http://www.newworldencyclopedia.org/entry/Alexander_Fleming

59. https://www.amymyersmd.com/2017/11/antibiotics-wreak-havoc-gut/

60. https://www.sciencedaily.com/releases/2013/01/130109081145.htm

61. https://www.amymyersmd.com/2017/11/antibiotics-wreak-havoc-gut/

62. https://drmasley.com/are-antibiotics-making-you-fat/

63. https://www.ncbi.nlm.nih.gov/pmc/articles/PMC5354595/

64. http://www.sustainabletable.org/257/antibiotics

65. https://drmasley.com/are-antibiotics-making-you-fat/

66. http://www.pamf.org/teen/health/nutrition/fastfood.html

67. http://www.back2normalpt.com/wp-content/uploads/2013/11/4_Toxicity-and-Food-Sensitivity_Oct-2013.pdf

68. https://draxe.com/glyphosate-in-cereal/?rs_oid_rd=668911093957143&utm_campaign=20180829_week35_curated_product&utm_medium=email&utm_source=smart+blast

69. https://www.psychologytoday.com/us/blog/ulterior-motives/201008/what-does-advertising-do

70. http://www.basicknowledge101.com/subjects/brain.html

71. http://drdavidhamilton.com/does-your-brain-distinguish-real-from-imaginary/

Part II

1. https://www.statista.com/topics/1244/physicians/

2. https://www.medicaldaily.com/average-woman-spends-17-years-her-life-diets-242601

3. https://www.completenutrition.com/blog/why-am-i-feeling-moody-while-dieting/

4. https://nutritionj.biomedcentral.com/articles/10.1186/1475-2891-10-9

5. https://www.medicaldaily.com/average-woman-spends-17-years-her-life-diets-242601

6. http://www.dailymail.co.uk/health/article-430913/Average-woman-spends-31-years-diet-researchers-say.html

7. https://www.glamour.com/story/shocking-body-image-news-97-percent-of-women-will-be-cruel-to-their-bodies-today

8. https://www.ncbi.nlm.nih.gov/pubmed/26178720

9. https://www.livestrong.com/article/392832-does-not-eating-slow-your-metabolism/

10. https://www.medicaldaily.com/average-woman-spends-17-years-her-life-diets-242601

11. https://www.webmd.com/vitamins/ai/ingredientmono-979/caffeine

12. https://www.mayoclinic.org/diseases-conditions/diabetes/expert-answers/artificial-sweeteners/faq-20058038

13. http://www.thedoctorwillseeyounow.com/content/dieting/art4151.html

14. https://www.medicalnewstoday.com/articles/261179.php

15. https://metro.co.uk/2016/12/30/how-long-does-it-take-to-change-a-habit-6351291/

16. https://metro.co.uk/2016/12/30/how-long-does-it-take-to-change-a-habit-6351291/

17. https://www.femalefirst.co.uk/health/length-of-the-average-diet-279944.html

18. https://www.optibacprobiotics.co.uk/live-cultures/articles/history-of-probiotics

19. Raw cheese is cheese made with unpasteurized milk. The good bacteria in these cheeses form a protective shield against potentially harmful contaminants, which means cheese made from raw milk may be healthier to consume than pasteurized cheese. https://www.pccmarkets.com/sound-consumer/2008-01/sc0801-cheese/.

20. https://www.medicalnewstoday.com/articles/319728.php

21. https://www.everydayhealth.com/columns/johannah-sakimura-nutrition-sleuth/need-lose-weight-just-add-fiber/

22. https://www.medicinenet.com/fiber/article.htm#fiber_for_bowel_disorders

23. https://www.medicinenet.com/fiber/article.htm#fiber_for_preventing_heart_disease

24. https://www.myfooddata.com/articles/fruits-high-in-fiber.php

25. https://en.wikipedia.org/wiki/Economics_of_coffee

26. https://www.thenakedscientists.com/articles/questions/can-i-reset-my-tolerance-caffeine

27. https://www.thenakedscientists.com/articles/questions/can-i-reset-my-tolerance-caffeine

28. https://www.teamiblends.com/best_ways_to_use_green_tea_for_

weight_loss

29. https://www.ncbi.nlm.nih.gov/pmc/articles/PMC3124776/

30. https://www.healthline.com/health/alcohol-and-weight-loss#alcohol-and-weight-loss

31. https://pubs.niaaa.nih.gov/publications/aa72/aa72.htm

32. http://time.com/28587/study-sugars-found-in-tequila-could-help-you-lose-weight/

33. https://www.quora.com/Is-protein-really-that-hard-to-digest

34. https://health.clevelandclinic.org/avoid-these-10-foods-full-of-trans-fats/

35. https://www.pcrm.org/health/health-topics/essential-fatty-acids

36. sugarscience.ucsf.edu/the-growing-concern-of-overconsumption.html

37. https://dtc.ucsf.edu/pdfs/calc-carbohydrates-by-food-weight.pdf

38. https://www.healthline.com/nutrition/18-most-addictive-foods#section1

39. https://nutritionj.biomedcentral.com/articles/10.1186/1475-2891-10-9

Other Sources

NV TECH. *The History of Vegetarianism.*
http://www.edu.pe.ca/sourishigh/Pages/Cmp6-03/Beth/Homepage/history_of_vegetarianism.htm>

Centers for Disease Control. Health, United States, 2016, table 53 [PDF – 9.8 MB]. https://www.cdc.gov/nchs/fastats/obesity-overweight.htm

ABC News. http://abcnews.go.com/Health/100-million-dieters-20-billion-weight-loss-industry/story?id=16297197

Bacon and Aphramor. "Evaluating the Evidence for a Paradigm Shift." BioMed Central. *Nutrition Journal* 201110:9, January 24, 2011. Ltd. 2011. https://doi.org/10.1186/1475-2891-10-9

About the Author

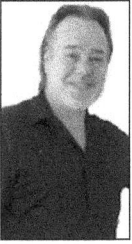

After earning his doctorate from NYCC in 1985 Dr. Rick Henningsen continued his post-graduate studies earning his certification as a Sports Physician, and a certification in Neuro-Electrodiagnostics. Proficient in numerous treatment modalities, diagnostic testing, imaging and functional impairment and disability ratings, Dr. Rick dedicated himself to the care and treatment of thousands of post traumatic injury patients for which weight loss played a key role as an adjunct to the course of treatment for many. Always seeking to improve the efficiency of patient treatment protocols, Dr. Rick organized multidisciplinary teams of allied health professionals, doctors, physicians and specialists to aid in providing the best care and treatment possible for his patients.

Following a career ending injury and subsequent surgery, Dr. Rick continued his commitment to improving the lives of others by tackling overweight and obesity, spending fifteen years in the hands-on research and trials of some of the most commonly used weight loss and dieting strategies to find out what works, what doesn't and why, and what he discovered about weight loss and dieting, and more importantly, how you can fix it, is shared inside *A Cure 4 Dieting*.

On his time off he earned the title of International Best-Selling Author and became an award-winning inventor for his design of the first ergonomic multifunction cross-over extension brush receiving the 'Popular Mechanics Editor's Choice Award for Design and Innovation.'

Dr. Rick strongly believes there is always room for improvement, a better way to do things and is committed to improving upon that which is lacking and there couldn't be a more concerning issue to tackle than those facing dieters, and the growing overweight and obesity epidemic, and his work there has not only provided some long sought-after answers to questions, and solutions to problems which have plagued dieters for the better part of a century... It will likely change the way the world looks at weight loss and dieting forever.